Medical Professional Liability and the Delivery of Obstetrical Care

VOLUME II
An Interdisciplinary Review

Victoria P. Rostow
and
Roger J. Bulger, editors

Committee to Study Medical Professional Liability
and the Delivery of Obstetrical Care

Division of Health Promotion and
Disease Prevention

INSTITUTE OF MEDICINE

NATIONAL ACADEMY PRESS
Washington, D.C. 1989

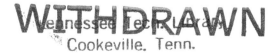

NATIONAL ACADEMY PRESS   2101 Constitution Avenue, NW   Washington, DC 20418

NOTICE: The papers in this volume were prepared as background material for the Institute of Medicine's Committee to Study Medical Professional Liability and the Delivery of Obstetrical Care. Most of the papers were presented at an interdisciplinary symposium held in Washington, D.C., on June 20, 1988. Support for the symposium and publication of this volume as a compendium to the committee's report was provided by the U.S. Department of Health and Human Services (Contract No. 282-88-0039).

The Institute of Medicine was chartered in 1970 by the National Academy of Sciences to enlist distinguished members of the appropriate professions in the examination of policy matters pertaining to the health of the public. In this, the Institute acts under both the Academy's 1863 congressional charter responsibility to be an adviser to the federal government and its own initiative in identifying issues of medical care, research, and education.

This project was supported by the Andrew W. Mellon Foundation contribution to the Institute of Medicine's (IOM) independent funds, the W.K. Kellogg Foundation contribution to IOM dissemination funds, the March of Dimes Birth Defects Foundation, and The Harris Foundation. The U.S. Department of Health and Human Services provided support for an interdisciplinary symposium and publication of background papers as the compendium volume to this report (Contract no. 282-88-0039).

Library of Congress Cataloging-in-Publication Data
(Revised for vol. II)
Institute of Medicine (U.S.). Committee to Study
  Medical Professional Liability and the Delivery of
  Obstetrical Care.
  Medical professional liability and the delivery of
obstetrical care.

  Vol. II contains background papers presented at an
interdisciplinary symposium held in Washington, D.C.,
on June 20, 1988.
  Bibliography: v. 1, p.
  Includes indexes.
  Contents: v. II. [without special title]—v. II. An
interdisciplinary review/Victoria P. Rostow and
Roger J. Bulger, editors.
  1. Obstetricians—Malpractice—United States.
2. Insurance, Physicians' liability—United States.
I. Rostow, Victoria P. II. Bulger, Roger J.,
1933–   . III. Title. [DNLM: 1. Insurance,
Liability—United States. 2. Malpractice—
United States. 3. Obstetrics—United States.
WP 33 AA1 I5m]
KF2910.G943157 1989   346.70303′32   89-12390
ISBN 0-309-03982-7 (v. I) 347.306332
ISBN 0-309-03986-X (v. II)

iii

Staff

VICTORIA P. ROSTOW, *Study Director,* Committee to Study Medical
Professional Liability and the Delivery of Obstetrical Care
ENRIQUETA C. BOND, *Executive Officer,* Institute of Medicine
MARIAN OSTERWEIS, *Acting Director,* Division of Health Promotion
and Disease Prevention
BOBBIE J. ALEXANDER, *Symposium Coordinator*
BLAIR POTTER, *Editor*

LIST OF CONTRIBUTORS

LORI ANDREWS, J.D., Research Fellow, American Bar Foundation, and Senior Scholar, Center for Clinical Medical Ethics, University of Chicago, Chicago

OTIS R. BOWEN, M.D., Former Secretary, U.S. Department of Health and Human Services, Washington, D.C.

ROGER J. BULGER, M.D., Chairman, Committee to Study Medical Professional Liability and the Delivery of Obstetrical Care, Institute of Medicine, and President, Association of Academic Health Centers, Washington, D.C.

SARAH D. COHN, C.N.M., J.D., Associate Counsel, Medicolegal Affairs, Yale-New Haven Hospital and Yale University, New Haven, Connecticut

STEPHEN DANIELS, Ph.D., Research Fellow, American Bar Foundation, Chicago

RICHARD A. EPSTEIN, LL.B., James Parker Hall Professor of Law, University of Chicago, and Editor, Journal of Legal Studies, Chicago

ELIZABETH H. ESTY, J.D., Associate, Sidley and Austin, Washington, D.C.

CYNTHIA FADER, B.S.N., Nurse, Labor and Delivery and Master's Candidate, Nurse-Midwifery, University of Pennsylvania, Philadelphia

JAMES A. HENDERSON, Jr., Frank B. Ingersoll Professor of Law, Cornell Law School, Ithaca, New York

NEIL A. HOLTZMAN, M.D., M.P.H., Professor, Department of Pediatrics, The Johns Hopkins University, Baltimore

DANA HUGHES, M.P.H., M.S., Senior Health Specialist, Children's Defense Fund, Washington, D.C.

DEBORAH LEWIS-IDEMA, M.Sc., Consultant, Health Policy and Planning, Washington, D.C.

W. HENSON MOORE, Partner, Sutherland, Asbill and Brennan, Washington, D.C.

CARTER G. PHILLIPS, J.D., Partner, Sidley and Austin, Washington, D.C.

ARNOLD RELMAN, M.D., Editor-in-Chief, The New England Journal of Medicine, and Professor of Medicine, Harvard Medical School, Cambridge, Massachusetts

SARA ROSENBAUM, J.D., Director, Child Health Division, The Children's Defense Fund, Washington, D.C.

VICTORIA P. ROSTOW, M.A., J.D., Study Director, Committee to Study Medical Professional Liability and the Delivery of Obstetrical Care, Institute of Medicine, Washington, D.C.

BENJAMIN P. SACHS, M.D., M.P.H., Associate Professor, Obstetrics and Gynecology, Harvard Medical School, and Associate Professor of Obstetrics and Gynecology, Harvard School of Public Health, Cambridge, Massachusetts

DAVID SMITH, J.D., Deputy Director, Division of Special Populations and Program Development, U.S. Department of Health and Human Services, Washington, D.C.

STEPHEN B. THACKER, M.D., M.Sc., Assistant Director for Science, Center for Environmental Health and Injury Control, Centers for Disease Control, Atlanta

Contents

EFFECTS ON ACCESS TO AND DELIVERY OF OBSTETRICAL CARE

THE LEGAL ISSUES

Preface

In October 1987 the Institute of Medicine (IOM) of the National Academy of Sciences appointed a distinguished interdisciplinary committee to evaluate the data relating to the effects of medical professional liability issues on access to and delivery of obstetrical care. Unlike many IOM reports that are undertaken at the request of Congress or of a government agency, this study was undertaken by the IOM on its own initiative following an inquiry by the American Academy of Pediatrics in 1984. The American Academy of Pediatrics, along with several other groups, believed that more attention to professional liability issues was urgently required. In addition, physicians, hospitals, insurers, and patients were becoming more and more vocal in their pleas for some solution to the problem of increasing numbers of claims, rising costs of jury verdicts and settlements, and higher medical malpractice insurance premiums. The IOM responded to this call.

What became known in many quarters as "the medical malpractice crisis" first came into focus in the mid-1970s. At that time, a series of studies reported that increasing numbers of medical malpractice suits, with ever higher awards, were prompting increases in medical malpractice insurance premiums and in some instances making medical malpractice insurance unavailable. At this same time, scholars from a variety of fields turned their attention to these issues, and several groups who were stakeholders in the medical malpractice controversy studied the problem and issued reports.

The fruits of this first phase of both scholarship and public policy debate on medical malpractice issues furnished the baseline for the IOM committee's data-gathering activities. By the time the IOM committee was in place in 1987, some facts had been established. First, research had confirmed that medical malpractice claims frequency and severity had increased throughout the decade. Second, 49 of 50 states had enacted major tort reforms since the mid-1970s. Consistent with this legislative activity, much of the literature produced during this period was concerned with the debate over reform of the tort system. Indeed, the IOM's own contribution to this debate, *Beyond Malpractice: Compensation for Medical Injuries,* which was published in 1978, developed a set of six criteria for evaluating tort reforms.

By 1987, however, it was clear that whatever momentum had been achieved in the last decade had been lost and that the debate on medical malpractice issues and reforms was at a standstill. The debate had become narrowly focused on tort reform. To be sure, a few scholars were advancing theoretical proposals setting forth alternatives to the tort system for compensating victims of injuries that occurred from medical malpractice. These alternative systems were debated in scholarly journals, but there had been little practical experience with them. Accordingly, in 1987 almost no data had been generated that would assist the IOM committee—or any other group—to evaluate the effectiveness of these proposals for imposing alternative regimes to resolve medical malpractice claims.

Moreover, some facts had changed in the decade since professional liability-related ills were first diagnosed as a problem for the American health care delivery system. By 1987 there was a new media focus on reports of obstetricians, family physicians, and nurse midwives who were abandoning obstetrical practice and thereby leaving certain segments of the population without adequate care. Yet although many individuals and groups readily accepted that professional liability issues posed a problem for the delivery of obstetrical care in the United States, little was known about the precise dimensions of the problem in practical terms or what to do about it. Indeed, the title for one of the General Accounting Office's 1986 reports to Congress on medical malpractice issues perhaps best summarizes the state of the policy debate at this time: *Medical Malpractice: No Agreement on the Problems or Solutions* (1986). It was against this background that the IOM committee began its work.

Early in its deliberations, the committee decided to focus its inquiry on access to and delivery of obstetrical care and to analyze various proposed solutions to the medical professional liability problem from the perspective of obstetrics, the field in which the problem was clearly most severe. Nationwide, obstetrics claims represent approximately 10 percent of all medical malpractice claims and nearly one-half of all indemnity payments. The committee also hoped that the case of obstetrics would prove an instructive vehicle for a study of the problems posed by professional liability issues for the health care system as a whole.

The committee quickly concluded that two things were required to move the public policy debate on the effects of medical professional liability in obstetrics toward a productive resolution. First, it believed that a consensus regarding the practical dimensions of the problem itself must be achieved. Second, it recognized that various options for solving the problem must be identified and assessed. The committee interpreted its mandate as the fulfillment of these two objectives.

From the outset the committee believed that its highly interdisciplinary composition was its major strength and its comparative advantage in relation to other individuals, groups, and organizations that have examined the question of professional liability in obstetrics. Accordingly, in approaching its task the committee tried to be as far-reaching as possible and to direct its efforts across whatever fields and disciplines were relevant to the problem.

As part of its data collection effort, the committee held an interdisciplinary symposium on June 20, 1988. The symposium, which was funded by the U.S. Department of Health and Human Services, featured fourteen noted scholars who were asked by the committee to turn their attention to certain problems related to the impact of professional liability issues on access to obstetrical care and on the way obstetrical care is delivered in the United States. In addition, four eminent legal scholars were asked to evaluate several recent legislative efforts to address the problems caused by professional liability issues in obstetrics and to set forth their ideas for resolving these questions. Otis R. Bowen, who was then secretary of the U.S. Department of Health and Human Services, gave the keynote address.

One of the committee's chief concerns was whether medical professional liability issues are affecting access to maternity care in the United States. The committee was particularly concerned with the effects of these issues on publicly financed obstetrical care because the women receiving such care are frequently both high-risk patients and underserved by the health care system.

Because community health centers are such an important source of obstetrical care for low-income women, the committee commissioned a survey of the effects of medical professional liability issues on the delivery of care in these centers. The results of that survey of a random sample of 208 Community and Migrant Health Center directors during April and May 1988 are presented in a paper by Dana Hughes, Sara

Rosenbaum, David Smith, and Cynthia Fader. The vast majority of these centers reported that medical professional liability concerns are either directly or indirectly compromising their ability to provide maternity care to poor women.

Yet community health centers represent only a small portion of the health care furnished to low-income women. The committee was equally concerned with women whose care is financed by Medicaid and with the problems of women who live in rural areas. The committee commissioned studies of both of these issues by Debra Lewis-Idema. The results of her investigation are startling. In her evaluation of approximately 40 state surveys, Ms. Lewis-Idema found that physicians are reporting that because of professional liability concerns they are curtailing their practices, limiting their Medicaid participation, and avoiding "high risk" patients who are very often socioeconomically disadvantaged women, poor women, and Medicaid women. She also found that medical professional liability concerns are creating significant access problems in rural areas, particularly among family physicians who provide two-thirds of the obstetrical care in rural areas.

The number of births attended by nurse-midwives in the United States, a provider group that is especially important to low-income and rural women, has increased substantially in recent years. The committee was troubled by reports that professional liability issues—the high cost and unavailability of medical malpractice insurance—were impairing the ability of nurse-midwives to deliver obstetrical care. Accordingly, it asked Sarah D. Cohn to address the question of the effects of medical professional liability issues on the delivery of obstetrical care by nurse-midwives. Her study makes it clear that the continued ability of nurse-midwives to furnish obstetrical care depends crucially on resolving the threat that medical professional liability issues pose for this group of obstetrical providers.

The question of how medical professional liability issues are affecting the actual practice of obstetrics also concerned the committee. The use of the electronic fetal monitor, the increase in cesarean section deliveries, and the development of technologies to screen for genetic disorders and birth defects offered instructive case studies to explore this question. Stephen B. Thacker presents a thorough study of electronic fetal monitoring, a technology whose use is believed to be at least partially driven by professional liability concerns. Similarly, many have alleged that professional liability concerns are driving the increase in the cesarean section rate, which has increased from 5 percent in the late 1960s to more than 25 percent in many urban areas today. Benjamin P. Sachs presents a scholarly examination of the many medical, legal, epidemiological, and social issues relevant to this growing practice. Neil A.

Holtzman examines how professional liability issues are shaping the development of technology for screening genetic disorders and birth defects and the legal issues that arise in applying these technologies. The most significant change in the practice of obstetrics, however, is also the most subtle and most difficult to support with data: the profound alteration in the physician-patient relationship that has been wrought by professional liability issues and the implications of this shift for patient care. These questions were addressed for the committee by Arnold Relman.

Although several studies, such as those undertaken by the General Accounting Office, have evaluated closed medical malpractice insurance claims, the committee believed that it was also important to study the subset of claims that actually proceed to court. As Stephen Daniels and Lori Andrews explain in their analysis of 24,625 civil verdicts from state trial courts of general jurisdiction in 46 counties in 11 states for the years 1981 to 1985: "The importance of jury verdicts lies not in their numbers, but in their symbolic value as 'transmitters of signals rather than as deciders of cases.'"

Finally, four noted legal scholars assessed some major proposals to reform the legal system that are particularly relevant to the problems posed by professional liability issues in obstetrics. Although the committee studied a wide range of possible solutions, the limits of time permitted at-length discussion of only four of these at the symposium: contractual solutions, administrative systems to adjudicate medical malpractice claims, limited no-fault insurance schemes for certain obstetrical injuries (a variant of what are known as Designated Compensable Events, or DCE, systems), and a proposal for a system of economic damage guarantees.

Various commentators have suggested replacing tort remedies for medical malpractice injuries with ex ante contractual agreements between physicians and patients that would set forth mutually agreeable processes to determine compensation should an injury occur. The committee, however, found that contractual solutions to medical professional liability issues are commonly misunderstood. Accordingly, it asked Richard A. Epstein to evaluate this approach and assess its appropriateness for obstetrical liability issues.

In 1987 the American Medical Association (AMA) unveiled an ambitious proposal to replace the civil justice system with a fault-based administrative system for resolving medical malpractice claims. At the request of the committee, Carter G. Phillips and Elizabeth H. Esty analyzed the implications of the AMA model from the perspective of obstetrical liability issues. In the past two years both Virginia and Florida have enacted statutes that provide no-fault compensation to certain neurologically impaired infants. These legislative remedies are designed to take these claims—which account for a significant proportion of the indemnity payments in most states—out of the civil justice system. The committee asked James A. Henderson, Jr. to evaluate this approach. Finally, W. Henson Moore, who introduced federal legislation in the 89th Congress to implement a variant of the economic damages guarantee system, discussed a variety of legislative options to resolve the professional liability problem in obstetrics.

The symposium attracted national attention. It was covered by more than a dozen newspapers, and segments were broadcast by two television networks. Not only were the media interested, but there was concern among legislators as well. On June 21, 1988, Roger J. Bulger and Victoria P. Rostow reported on the committee's preliminary findings to the U.S. Congress's Joint Economic Committee.

We hope that this companion volume to the committee's report will prove valuable to scholars, policy analysts, legislators, and legislative analysts, as well as to students of law, medicine, public policy, and public health, as they endeavor to understand and resolve the problems posed by medical professional liability issues to the delivery of health care in America.

VICTORIA P. ROSTOW
ROGER J. BULGER

Medical Professional Liability and the Delivery of Obstetrical Care

An Interdisciplinary Review

Keynote Address

OTIS R. BOWEN, M.D.

The growing cost of medical malpractice insurance and the impact it is having on people's access to prenatal care and delivery services is a problem of profound importance to this country.

I want to thank the Institute of Medicine for its leadership in attacking this problem. In doing so, it is building on the work of a U.S. Department of Health and Human Services (HHS) task force I convened a couple of years ago to investigate the impact that growing medical liability and malpractice costs are having on people's access to health care. That task force discovered that the hardest hit of all medical services was obstetrics.

From 1982 to 1985 the average malpractice insurance premium for all physicians increased by 81 percent, whereas rates for obstetrician-gynecologists shot up 113 percent. A growing response of obstetricians and family physicians to these skyrocketing premium costs has been to curtail or omit delivery services altogether. Just last year the American Academy of Family Physicians reported that 18.6 percent of its members have dropped their obstetrical practice, giving as their reason either liability insurance costs or an inability to get malpractice insurance.

Obstetrician-gynecologists (ob-gyns) in particular also fear malpractice suits—and small wonder. More than 73 percent report that they have been sued at least once. Verdicts or settlements for obstetrical cases can be in the million-dollar range, a figure that does not even count the hefty legal costs involved.

1

These factors in turn have helped to send insurance premiums soaring for ob-gyns. A survey conducted by the American College of Obstetricians and Gynecologists showed that the average premium for their members' liability insurance went from nearly $11,000 in 1982 to more than $37,000 in 1987—more than a threefold increase.

Two groups of patients have felt the greatest impact from these changes: those living in rural areas and those with low incomes living in the inner cities. A physician has to deliver about 40 babies nowadays just to cover the cost of one year's malpractice premium, but the fact is that many rural doctors are not called on to make that many deliveries. With family physicians often the only ones to serve an area, numerous counties or entire regions of some states report that they have just one or two physicians to deliver babies.

Informal surveys tell this story all too well:

• By early 1987, Arizona's rural counties reported a 30 percent drop in obstetrical providers during the previous three years.

• In Alabama, 300 of 441 family physicians responding to a 1986 survey had stopped practicing obstetrics.

• In Mississippi a survey of family physicians was no more reassuring: in 1985, 35 percent of them included maternity care in their practice; by 1987, the number had fallen to 14 percent.

• A Texas Medical Association study in 1987 found that 69 percent of all Texas family and general practitioners had limited or eliminated some of the services they were providing; 37 percent had discontinued their obstetrical practice altogether.

Another group of maternity care providers has also been hard hit by the increases in malpractice insurance rates—those who serve in federally funded Community Health Centers. These centers serve Medicaid recipients and other low-income patients in medically underserved rural and inner-city areas. A significant part of their service is maternity care. These centers face increased liability insurance costs because so many of the young women they serve are at special risk. Having to pay higher rates puts these centers in a particularly tight financial bind, for two reasons: (1) they cannot pass the increased cost on to their low-income patients, and (2) there are limits on the federal funds they receive. Some states have increased Medicaid payments for maternity care, although nearly all such payments remain far below physicians' usual charges and private insurance rates.

All of these problems stand in the way of the special initiative the HHS has under way to drive down infant mortality rates in this country. This initiative was undertaken because the steady decline in the nation's infant mortality rate showed signs of slowing down. (As a nation the United States' rate is still well above those of many industrialized countries.) In fact, there does not appear to be any change in the incidence of low-birthweight babies; there has even been a slight increase in the percentage of very low birthweight infants.

There is even less room for optimism in another key indicator: the percentage of women in the first trimester of pregnancy who are receiving prenatal care. We found no increase in this percentage. I need hardly elaborate on how vital early prenatal care is to driving down infant mortality rates. It is, quite simply, a key to all our efforts and offers us the best hope of success.

Much credit has been given to the development of neonatal intensive care units in the overall effort to save infants born with life-threatening conditions. The men and women who work in these units deserve our highest praise for their lifesaving work. They are writing a lustrous new chapter in the annals of medicine. Still, as we give these heroes our praise, there is a point to be made that they would be among the first to assert: neonatal intensive care is frightfully expensive. Bills of $30,000 and more are not uncommon in an effort to save a single infant. Even when the infant is saved, it very often faces an uncertain future with considerable impediments to its health and functioning. Saving infants to live a life of nearly total dependency poses agonizing choices for parents and sometimes puts them at odds with the men and women of neonatal intensive care units whose jobs are to save infants' lives.

All of these factors drive thoughtful people to reflect on how much better it would be to ensure that all pregnant women received high-quality prenatal care, which can often help to avoid these agonizing choices by ensuring that fewer infants are born with intractable, life-long medical problems. A $30,000 neonatal intensive care bill could easily cover the costs of high-quality prenatal care for many women throughout their pregnancy. In a nation like ours, in which soaring health care bills are a problem all their own, this is no small consideration.

The blunt fact is that this country must find less expensive ways of ensuring the good health of its people or face the dismal prospect of a health care system in which the voracious demands of high-technology medicine will preempt the nation's capacity to provide access to care for increasing numbers of its people. Some 37 million Americans today are without any financial coverage for their health care. At least 17 percent of women in their childbearing years have no insurance at all, and between 11 and 12 million children are without health insurance coverage.

If we are to reverse this dangerous state of affairs, we simply must find ways of ensuring sound health care for more people at an affordable cost.

We can only accomplish that goal by redirecting our health care system so that it puts greater emphasis on low-cost prevention rather than high-cost technology.

I am not an enemy of high-technology medicine. The danger I see today, however, is that high-tech medicine will become its own worst enemy. If its cost becomes too high, we will see public and private insurers putting arbitrary restrictions on its use. That kind of action is rationing, and we certainly do not want that. We want a system that uses the technology that is most appropriate to the individual situation, but there is absolutely no hope of achieving that desirable state of affairs if physicians keep dropping out of maternal and obstetrical care.

Two of our chief enemies in this instance are fear and ignorance. Physicians fear being sued, and the system lacks the knowledge it needs to defend physicians from suits that are based more on emotion than on fact. Physicians feel themselves to be at the mercy of juries of nonmedical people whose sympathies may often rest with parents and babies. To counteract this all too human tendency, physicians need a body of widely accepted knowledge about what constitutes legally defensible obstetrical practice.

Unfortunately, no such body of knowledge exists. We urgently need data that will allow us to see more precisely the relationship between what course of treatment or procedure the physician elects and the likely outcome for a mother and her infant.

The department's National Center for Health Services Research and Health Care Technology Assessment is at work on this problem on a broader scale. Researchers there believe—and I agree—that carefully selected studies of patient outcomes can offer us two considerable advantages: (1) they can improve the quality of patient care, and (2) they can serve to reduce unwarranted malpractice suits.

The final report of my Task Force on Medical Liability and Malpractice set forth six important public policy issues that research can help us resolve:

• First, we need to know the frequency of adverse medical outcomes and how we can distinguish between avoidable and unavoidable results.

• Second, we need to know the relationship between physician practice patterns and malpractice claims. In this regard a national data bank being set up by HHS will give us information on malpractice claims and licensure actions, as well as permit interstate comparisons.

• Third, we need to know what kinds of actions are effective in preventing substandard practices among physicians. I am referring to such mechanisms as state licensure boards and the work of peer review organizations.

- Fourth, we need to know how the quality of care is affected by hospital risk management programs, the practice of defensive medicine, and the use of innovative medical technology.
- Fifth, we need to know how effective various tort reforms are in stemming the tide of malpractice suits and what many regard as excessive monetary settlements.
- Sixth, we need to know more about the insurance system itself. What factors are at work in the industry that affect the cost of professional liability and insurance underwriting practice?

The studies will help us find answers to these important policy questions. For example, HHS has a research program mandated by 1986 legislation that is looking into variations in medical practice. It is designed to provide clinicians and those who buy health care with the costs and value of alternative practices and procedures. In addition the Public Health Service has convened an expert panel on the content of prenatal care. These kinds of efforts can help tell us what is appropriate medical practice today and what is not. To the extent that they do, they can help reduce our reliance on the courts to solve issues of medical malpractice.

That about concludes my remarks, except for one thing: there is a tendency at times to think that Washington has all the answers to our society's problems. The simple truth is that Washington did not create all of the problems and it is not going to solve all of them. I believe the federal government has a role to play in the issue before this symposium, but I believe that others among us have equally important roles. This symposium is in fact a simple acknowledgment of that view. Other professional organizations in medicine have a stake in this question, and they have become involved in the quest for answers. The states have entered the arena, too. When I was governor of Indiana, I helped steer to passage medical malpractice legislation that has made a significant dent in Indiana's problem. Other states have also acted. A few have addressed the specific problems that rising obstetrical malpractice rates have brought on them.

- Virginia enacted a Birth-Related Neurological Injury Compensation Act in response to a statewide crisis in the availability and cost of insurance for obstetricians.
- Missouri now has a law requiring the state to cover malpractice awards against physicians who provide obstetric and pediatric services in public clinics.
- Hawaii has created a state fund to help cover liability insurance premiums so that those who provide obstetrical services will be induced to practice in underserved areas of the state.

We must each continue to do our part to solve this problem—or I should say "problems," because what we are facing is the result of many factors that will demand many kinds of solutions. Above all, we must share with each other our findings and perspectives. Viable, long-lasting solutions will be found only when all of us work together—government at all levels, medicine, the legal profession, and the insurance industry—to get command of the facts and find out what really works.

This symposium is a good step in that direction—and now, let its real work begin, for the children's sake.

The Medical Background

The Impact of Technology Assessment and Medical Malpractice on the Diffusion of Medical Technologies: The Case of Electronic Fetal Monitoring

STEPHEN B. THACKER, M.D., M.SC.

In this chapter I address several topics related to electronic fetal monitoring (EFM), a procedure used in labor to detect fetal distress. First, I describe EFM and give an overview of the history of its use in the United States. I then focus on the evidence for its efficacy and safety and discuss the impact on clinical practice of current policies and emerging research findings. Finally, I use the history of EFM to describe the diffusion of technology and the policies that affect diffusion, and to discuss in particular the impact of technology assessment and medical malpractice on the diffusion of technology.

HISTORY OF FETAL MONITORING

The status of the fetus during labor has been monitored for centuries. In fact listening to the fetal heart rate through a stethoscope (auscultation) has been a part of labor management for more than 100 years. Fetal bradycardia (abnormally slow heart rate) and meconium staining of amniotic fluid were recognized as indicators of fetal distress in the late nineteenth century.[1] Attempts to record the fetal heart rate (FHR) began as early as 1891; however, current electronic methods of fetal monitoring have been developed since 1960.

Use of trade names is for identification only and does not constitute endorsement by the Public Health Service or the U.S. Department of Health and Human Services.

In 1957 Hon first reported the successful recording of the fetal electro-cardiogram (EKG) from the mother's abdomen.[2] In 1959 he observed profound bradycardia in a dying fetus and noted that manipulation of the prolapsed cord caused cardiac irregularities and bradycardia.[3] In 1960 Hon described a clinical FHR monitor, although he recognized the need for a better method of recording.[4] According to Hehre, Hon conceived the idea of passing an electrode through the cervix and clipping it to the fetus's head to record the EKG; he made a prototype of the device in his home workshop and appeared for the initial testing of it in the delivery room at 3 a.m.[5] The electrode was successful and became the basis for present EFM devices; a major improvement, the spiral electrode, was developed by Hon in 1972.[6]

By 1969, EFM by ultrasound and by direct EKG monitoring had begun to diffuse rapidly. Hon and Caldeyro-Barcia were the most active investigators, describing a variety of changes in the FHR and correlating them with clinical status. Working independently, these two men devised different schemes for interpreting FHR patterns. Because of the resulting confusion in the obstetrical community, they agreed on a standard terminology in the 1970s.[7]

In 1961 Saling reported a technique for sampling fetal scalp-blood.[8] In this technique a scalpel is passed through the cervical os, and a small wound is made in the baby's scalp. A sample of blood is then collected in a capillary tube and analyzed for acid–base parameters, pH being the most widely accepted measure of fetal well-being. This technique has gradually come to be considered an integral part of EFM and is often used to validate a diagnosis made by FHR monitoring.

At first, EFM was used largely for high-risk pregnancies, and some physicians continue to advocate its use primarily for that group. An increasing number of obstetricians, however, favor EFM during all labors, and many institutions in this country and elsewhere use it routinely. By 1972 an estimated 1,000 EFM systems were in use in the United States, and a survey in 1976 reported that 278 of 279 obstetrics programs with residencies in obstetrics used EFM.[9] Surveys of physicians reported in 1970 and 1976 found a high degree of acceptance of the procedure, and the 1976 survey showed that 77 percent of the physicians surveyed believed that EFM should be used in all labors.[10, 11]

Today, EFM is done externally (using ultrasound), internally (by attaching electrodes directly to the fetus to monitor its EKG), or sequentially (using both techniques before and after the amniotic sac ruptures). For internal monitoring, a catheter is used to monitor uterine contractions.

Despite the widespread application of EFM and an extensive literature on the interpretation of results, there is surprisingly little data on its pattern of use in the community. Several reports have described patterns of use at individual institutions, however. Initial reports from several university or large teaching programs demonstrated that clinicians attempted to use EFM for all labors within two years of purchasing a monitor. At these institutions, the percentage of pregnancies for which EFM was used ranged from 86 to 100.[12] Later reports indicated less widespread monitoring at community-based institutions.

Few population-based studies have been performed. One based on 1978 birth records from upstate New York, however, found that 47 percent of live births had some form of electronic monitoring, with external EFM predominating.[13] Data from the 1980 National Natality Survey were almost identical: EFM was used in 47.7 percent of live births, and EFM predominated.[14] By 1986, 75 percent of live births in New York State were monitored electronically, most of them externally (D. Mayack, personal communication, 1988). The National Natality Survey will include detailed questions about EFM when it is reported in 1990 (P. Placek, personal communication, 1988).

Advocates of EFM promised that its use would reduce the rate of intrapartum stillbirth, neonatal illness and death, and developmental disabilities. Early, uncontrolled observations showed a reduction in both perinatal mortality and low Apgar scores in association with the increased use of EFM during labor. Moreover, labors monitored with EFM had superior outcomes compared with other, less complicated labors without EFM in the same institution. Nonetheless, widespread introduction of this technology prompted national controversy in the 1970s, controversy that was heightened after four randomized clinical trials indicated little or no benefit with EFM.[15] Reports of five additional clinical trials have been published—all but one with negative results— yet established policies for intrapartum surveillance with EFM have not been altered as a result.[16, 17] Although the controversy surrounding EFM has diminished substantially during the 1980s, the proper role of EFM in intrapartum care has not been settled.

EFFICACY AND SAFETY OF ELECTRONIC FETAL MONITORING

Technology assessment is the systematic study of the possible effects on society of new, extended, or modified technology, with special emphasis on impacts that are unintended, indirect, and delayed.[18] The assessment's purpose is to provide decision makers with information on policy alternatives, such as allocating research and development funds, formulating regulations, or developing new legislation. The ultimate goal of technology assessment, however, is to improve outcome.

The congressional Office of Technology Assessment took the lead in technology assessment in the United States in the 1970s, and now interest and activities are widespread in government, universities, and the private sector. At the Institute of Medicine, the Council on Health Care Technology addresses central issues in technology assessment through panels on information, methods, and evaluation.

The basic task of technology assessment is to document efficacy and safety. The key tool in the evolution of efficacy is the randomized clinical trial (RCT). Primary clinical evaluations can be ranked according to their freedom from bias: RCTs appear at the top, followed by nonrandomized controlled studies, series of patients without controls, and personal recollection unaided by systematic recordkeeping. Yet with the notable exception of drug trials, RCTs are rarely conducted before a technology has been diffused. Because of their expense, limited generalizability, and difficulty of implementation, RCTs rarely provide sufficient evidence to encourage or limit the diffusion of a new technology or to necessitate the withdrawal of a widely used technology. A thorough technology assessment is expensive and time-consuming and is simply not practical for all medical technologies. Even when well conducted, the findings may be overridden by social, economic, or political considerations.

None of the nine RCTs noted in the last section demonstrated a statistically significant decrease with the use of EFM in the rates of perinatal death, intrapartum stillbirth, neonatal death, 1-minute Apgar score of < 7, 1-minute Apgar score of < 4, or neonatal intensive care admissions (Table 1). The first Melbourne trial and the second Denver trial showed a decrease in neonatal seizures associated with EFM and the use of fetal scalp-blood sampling.[19, 20] Whereas the decrease was not statistically significant, this observation confirmed the finding in the Dublin study.[21] The first Melbourne study suggested a significant decrease associated with EFM in the rate of admission to neonatal intensive care units, associated with EFM, a finding not confirmed elsewhere. All of the trials showed an increased rate of cesarean delivery in the EFM group. The results for total operative deliveries were mixed: increases in the rates of operative deliveries (that is, abdominal and forceps deliveries) were reported in the EFM group in both Melbourne trials, the second Denver trial, and both the Copenhagen and Dublin studies; decreases were reported in the EFM group in the first Denver and the Sheffield trials.[22-28]

The pooled data* showed slight but not significant increases in the EFM group in the number of low Apgar scores, the number of admissions

---

*Because the Dallas study was designed to compare the results of hospital policies that related to the restricted availability of EFM rather than the use of EFM compared with auscultation, I did not pool these data.[29]

to neonatal intensive care units, and the perinatal death rate (Table 2). The EFM group did, however, show a statistically significant decrease in the number of neonatal seizures. It also had statistically significant increases in the rate of both abdominal and total operative deliveries.

A review of only those RCTs that involved high-risk pregnancies shows nonsignificant increases in the EFM group in the rates of perinatal death and of infants with Apgar scores of < 7 and nonsignificant decreases in the rates of neonatal seizures and admission to neonatal intensive care units. A statistically significant doubling of the rate of cesarean delivery was evident in the EFM group, however, and total operative deliveries were increased in high-risk pregnancies.

In pooling data from the trials in which fetal scalp-blood sampling was used to complement electronic monitoring, I found lower but statistically significant increases in the rates of cesarean delivery and total operative deliveries in the EFM group. The rate of neonatal seizure, on the other hand, decreased twofold when fetal scalp-blood sampling was used to complement electronic monitoring, although without the large Dublin trial this decrease is not statistically significant.

These findings leave pregnant women, as well as physicians and midwives, in a dilemma. Is preventing potentially serious but uncommon events (e.g., neonatal seizures) worth the much higher risk of operative delivery? The long-term clinical implications of seizures remain unclear. Published reports indicate that neonatal seizures are a serious prognostic finding; yet follow-up of the 39 Dublin infants with seizures who survived the neonatal period shows no difference in the outcomes for the auscultation and EFM groups at 1 year of age.[30] This finding suggests that more sensitive diagnostic criteria may have been used in the Dublin trial or that seizures with adverse prognostic implications are not affected by early intervention during labor and delivery. Investigators in the Dublin trial analyzed their data and found that the benefits of EFM were restricted to an association with protracted labor and with women given oxytocin (to induce or speed up labor). Although appropriately cautious about overanalyzing their data, they state that selective use of EFM may be preferable to universal use. The use of selective monitoring was tested in the Dallas and Seattle trials, but investigators found no measurable benefit to this approach, at least with their particular sets of selection criteria.[31, 32]

Establishing policy in clinical practice requires not only determining whether a screening procedure is effective but also determining whether the human and monetary costs are acceptable. Moreover, the effectiveness, safety, and acceptability of subsequent interventions must be considered. For example, the evidence reviewed here demonstrates a significant increase in the rate of operative deliveries associ-

TABLE 1 Results of Nine Clinical Trials Assessing the Efficacy of Routine Electronic Fetal Monitoring During Labor

Characteristic	Denver 1976 E-I	A	Melbourne 1976 E-II	A	Sheffield 1978 E-I	A	Denver 1979 E-I	E-II	A	Melbourne 1981 E-II	A	Copenhagen 1981 E-II	A	Dublin 1985 E-II	A	Dallas 1986 U	S	Seattle 1987 E-II	A
Subjects																			
Pregnant women	242	241	175	175	253	251	233	230	232	445	482	482	487	6,474	6,490	17,586	17,409	124	124
Infants	242	241	175	175	253	251	233	230	232	445	482	485	493	6,530	6,554	17,759	17,571	122	124
Maternal risk status	High		High		Low		High			Low		All[a]		All[b]		All		High	
Fetal scalp-blood sampling	No	—	Yes	—	No	—	No	Yes	—	Yes	—	Yes	—	Yes	—	No	—	Yes	—
Cesarean deliveries																			
Total	40	16	39	24	24	11	41	26	13	18	10	28	18	158	144	1,933	1,777	19	19
Percentage	16.5	6.6	22.3	13.7	9.5	4.4	17.6	11.3	5.6	5.8	2.7	5.7	3.7	2.4	2.2	11.0	10.2	15.6	15.2
With fetal distress	18	3	16	9	4	3	16	8	1	NA	NA	8	7	25	10	454	369	10	7
Percentage	7.4	1.2	9.1	5.1	1.6	1.2	6.9	3.5	0.4	NA	NA	1.6	1.4	0.4	0.2	2.6	2.1	8.2	5.6
Operative vaginal deliveries																			
Number	60	78	70	67	71	78	64	54	54	120	101	85	64	528	407	NA	NA	NA	NA
Percentage	24.8	32.4	40.0	38.3	28.1	31.1	27.5	23.5	23.3	27.0	20.7	17.6	13.1	8.2	6.3	NA	NA	NA	NA
1-Minute Apgar score < 7																			
Number	31	29	28	25	24	24	41	35	33	39	40	28	32	216[c]	227[c]	NA	NA	NA	NA
Percentage	12.8	12.0	16.0	14.3	9.6	9.5	17.5	15.2	14.2	8.3	8.8	5.8	6.5	4.3	4.5	NA	NA	NA	NA
1-Minute Apgar score < 4																			

Number	NA	NA	4	6	4	7	14	10	11	4	6	5	7	62	57	NA	NA	38	35
Percentage	NA	NA	2.3	3.4	1.6	2.8	6.0	4.3	4.7	0.9	1.2	1.0	1.4	1.0	0.9	NA	NA	31	28
Neonatal seizures																			
Number	2	2	0	4	0	1	2	0	2	0	0	0	0	12	27	53	45	7	7
Rate per 1,000	8.3	8.3	0.0	22.9	0.0	4.0	8.6	0.0	8.6	0.0	0.0	0.0	0.0	1.8	4.1	3.0	2.6	5.7	5.7
Total receiving oxytocin	NA	NA	0	NA	0	NA	NA	0	NA	0	0	0	0	4	19	NA	NA	NA	NA
Neonatal intensive care No. of admissions	35	28	11	30	45	43	23	29	29	59	48	51	49	547	543	460	428	NA	NA
Percentage	14.5	11.6	6.3	17.1	17.8	17.1	9.9	12.6	12.5	13.3	10.0	10.5	9.9	8.4	8.3	2.6	2.5	NA	NA
Mean length of stay (days)	NA	NA	3.1[d]	3.8[d]	NA	NA	NA	NA	NA	NA	NA	4.0	5.7	NA	NA	NA	NA	NA	NA
Perinatal deaths Rate per 1,000	8.3	4.1	5.7	5.7	0.0	4.0	8.6	4.3	0.0	2.2	0.0	0.0	2.1	2.1	2.1	14.8	17.0	139	145
Stillbirths	0	0	0	1	0	0	0	0	0	0	0	0	1	3	2	148	186	NA	NA
Neonatal deaths	2	1	1	0	0	1	2	1	0	1	0	0	0	11	12	114	113	NA	NA

NOTE: E-I = group with electronic fetal monitoring only (experimental); E-II = group with electronic fetal monitoring and scalp-blood sampling (experimental); U = group with universal electronic fetal monitoring; S = group with selective fetal monitoring; A = auscultation group (control); NA = not available.

[a] Excludes women with diabetes mellitus; classes B, C, D, and F.
[b] Excludes women with abnormal amniotic fluid on admission.
[c] Data collected on first 10,094 pregnancies; complete on 10,035.
[d] Data could not be verified by author.

SOURCE: Thacker, S. B. 1987. The efficacy of intrapartum electronic fetal monitoring. Am. J. Obstet. Gynecol. 156:24-30; updated, 1988.

TABLE 2   Pooled Data from Eight Randomized, Controlled Trials of Electronic Fetal Monitoring

Measure	Pooled Relative Risk	95% Confidence Interval	Test for Heterogeneity
	Outcome		
Apgar score < 7	1.01	0.88–1.15	$x^2/8$ = 1.90 (NS)[a]
Apgar score < 4	1.02	0.80–1.30	$x^2/8$ = 2.71 (NS)
Neonatal seizure	0.52	0.32–0.84	$x^2/8$ = 5.66 (NS)
NICU admission[b]	1.01	0.84–1.21	$x^2/8$ = 14.18 (NS)
Perinatal death	1.17	0.62–2.19	$x^2/7$ = 9.73 (NS)
	Complication		
Cesarean delivery[c]	2.02	1.62–2.51	$x^2/7$ = 8.06 (NS)
Operative vaginal deliveries[c]	1.10	0.96–1.27	$x^2/6$ = 11.66 (NS)
Total operative deliveries	1.33	1.22–1.46	$x^2/7$ = 8.80 (NS)

NOTE: Because data for some of these outcomes were not available in all eight randomized trials, some of the pooled results are based on fewer trials. Unavailable data are noted in Table 1.

[a]NS = not statistically significant.

[b]NICU = neonatal intensive care unit.

[c]Because of a statistically significant increase in heterogeneity, results of the Dublin trial could not be pooled with cesarean deliveries and operative vaginal deliveries, but they are included in total operative deliveries.

SOURCE: Thacker, S. B. 1987. The efficacy of intrapartum electronic fetal monitoring. Am. J. Obstet. Gynecol. 156:24–30; updated, 1988.

ated with EFM, with or without fetal scalp-blood sampling. If used in essentially all pregnancies, EFM will have large, direct financial costs, and these costs will increase dramatically if EFM is associated with an intervention (for example, cesarean delivery) that may often be unnecessary. When a decision is made about the routine use of EFM, its value should be assessed in view of the potential benefit of alternative obstetrical practices designed to decrease perinatal morbidity and mortality. Knowing these alternatives helps pregnant women, physicians, and midwives understand the impact of their choices on both maternal and infant well-being.

DIFFUSION OF TECHNOLOGY

Diffusion refers to the spread of an innovation over time in a social system. The determinants of diffusion are complex. Fineberg[33] has identified 10 influences on diffusion: (1) prevailing theory, (2) benefits of the innovation, (3) features of the clinical situation, (4) presence of an advocate, (5) characteristics of the adoption, (6) practice setting, (7) channels of communication, (8) the decision-making process, (9) evaluation, and (10) environmental constraints.

The perceived importance of asphyxia as a cause of neonatal mortality and morbidity in the 1970s facilitated the diffusion of EFM. Further, the benefits to the physician were great: EFM was relatively easy to learn, imposed little change on practice style, and replaced a practice—intermittent auscultation—that was imperfect and dependent on the skills of the nursing staff. EFM addressed a problem of great concern at the time—perinatal mortality—and appeared during a period of wide acceptance of new technology. It had strong advocates who were well represented in the obstetrical community, both in the United States and internationally.

The potential users of EFM—clinicians—were led by their colleagues in academic centers, who were at the forefront of EFM use and who communicated their preference in medical journals and at professional meetings. Newly certified obstetricians were uncomfortable with intermittent auscultation because as house officers they had had little experience in using it. Decision making in medicine moves most quickly when practice decisions are made exclusively by the individual practitioner, which probably facilitated the rapid spread of EFM use in the United States. All of these influences in the case of EFM tended to facilitate its rapid diffusion into clinical practice.

The remaining two sources of influence—environmental constraints through regulatory agencies and medical care insurers and evaluation through technology assessment—are influenced more by policymakers than physicians. In the sections that follow I address specific policies for EFM, as well as the role of technology assessment in general.

Policies Toward Medical Technology

There are four stages in the development of a technology: (1) basic and applied research, (2) clinical trials to demonstrate efficacy and safety, (3) diffusion, and (4) widespread use. Programs have been developed to try to improve the process at each stage.[34] Thus, the National Institutes of Health (NIH) supports research, including some clinical trials; the Food and Drug Administration (FDA) requires companies to demonstrate efficacy and safety of medical devices before marketing; health planning agencies have some limited control over the diffusion of certain technologies; Medicare and Medicaid reimburse for the use of technologies that are determined to be medically necessary; and the Peer Review Organizations (PROs) review medical practice to ensure appropriate use.

The private sector is also involved at each stage of development and in some cases implements formal policies similar to those of the federal government. Each stage involves many complex interactions between the public and private sectors.

Policies Toward Development of Electronic Fetal Monitoring

The National Institutes of Health awarded to investigators at the University of Southern California (a major developer of EFM) almost $1 million in contracts for specific developmental research on EFM between 1971 and 1975. At the same time, Corometrics, one of the major manufacturers of EFM equipment, funded research at the University of Southern California, although published papers did not acknowledge that funding. This phenomenon of research funding by interest groups is common in medicine, but it is a source of bias that needs to be recognized.

Policies Toward Evaluation of Electronic Fetal Monitoring

In addition to its primary role in research and development, the NIH is the main supporter of technology evaluations. Grants from the NIH tend to be awarded to persons who have worked hard to develop a technology; yet these researchers, with their vested interest in the technology, are not the ideal choice to organize and carry out an impartial evaluation. This was certainly true with EFM, a case in which investigators at the University of Southern California had received a large amount of financial support to study patient series and carry out nonrandomized, controlled studies. The NIH did not, however, provide support for clinical trials to evaluate either EFM or fetal scalp-blood sampling: the two early randomized clinical trials of EFM in the United States were funded by the Maternal and Child Health Program of the Health Services Administration, U.S. Department of Health, Education, and Welfare (now the U.S. Department of Health and Human Services), which has a direct interest in ensuring the efficacy and safety of the services it supplies.[35, 36]

Recognizing the lack of validated information for many medical technologies, the NIH developed a "consensus" mechanism in which experts are brought together to examine available evidence and clinical experience and to make recommendations. A consensus group dealing with EFM released a draft report and held an open meeting in 1979.[37] It concluded that EFM is potentially beneficial in all pregnancies and that it should be strongly considered in high-risk pregnancies. At the same time, the consensus panel concluded that intermittent auscultation was acceptable for intrapartum monitoring in all pregnancies. This consensus mechanism, however, has been found to have little measurable impact on clinical practice.[38]

The Medical Devices Program was established by the Medical Devices Amendments of 1976.[39] Modeled after the Food and Drug Act, which regulates drugs, the amendments require the demonstration of "effectiveness" and safety before a device can be marketed. Using the FDA approach, companies wishing to market a medical device are required to present evidence, usually including the results of RCTs, showing effectiveness and safety before the device is approved for marketing.

Under the Medical Devices Amendments, all devices are classified by special panels into one of three groups, depending on the regulatory controls needed to provide reasonable assurance of their safety and effectiveness. Class I is general controls; class II, performance standards; and class III, premarket approval. Most devices now on the market will be in class II, depending on whether it is possible to develop performance standards to ensure safety and effectiveness.

These regulations focus on safety and pay little attention to efficacy or effectiveness. The FDA generally uses a definition of effectiveness that indicates that the drug or device must do what the manufacturer claims it will do. For drugs, this policy has meant that anticoagulants, for example, are evaluated for their ability to prevent coagulation and not for their ability to intervene in disease processes such as recurrent myocardial infarction. The use of the Food and Drug Act as a model for the Medical Devices Amendments implies that EFM devices will be evaluated on their ability, for example, to reliably record the fetal heart rate but may not be evaluated on whether accurate recording of the fetal heart rate makes any difference to the outcome of the infant. According to the FDA, no specific actions have been taken on EFM devices since the amendments were implemented (G. Johnson, personal communication, 1988).

Policies Toward Payment for Electronic Fetal Monitoring

If institutions that provide EFM were to include it as part of their obstetrical package, there would be no financial incentive to use EFM— there might even be a mild disincentive because it does have direct costs. If institutions charge separately for EFM, however, there is an incentive to use the equipment to recoup the investment. A survey of 563 institutions known to use EFM in 1975 revealed that 142 of the 344 respondents (46.3 percent) charged a separate fee, the most common being $25.[40]

Third-party payers, such as Blue Cross, generally reimburse institutions for their charges, depending on the specifics of the medical-care contract with the patient. Such reimbursement is generally available through insurance. The only major government program involved, the Medicaid program, generally follows the lead of Blue Cross and other major insurance programs. Thus, third-party payment for EFM is readily available.

Policies Toward Use of Electronic Fetal Monitoring

The only federal program that deals directly with technology use is that involving the Peer Review Organizations.[41] Most PROs are transformed Professional Standards Review Organizations, and although reviews are restricted to Medicare patients, PROs have been encouraged to enter into similar contracts with Medicaid and other third-party payers. The PRO program is a cost-control and quality-assurance program that reviews primarily hospital services. The law requires that PROs use norms, criteria, and standards in evaluating medical services. Standards are usually developed by a consensus of physicians, based on typical patterns of practice in the area and on such regional or national information as may be available; however, because the PRO is a peer review, physician-run program, standards have been largely local. Because there is strong support for EFM among practicing obstetricians, PROs probably could not be used to control EFM use.

Malpractice litigation is often the only recourse a patient has, and it offers a powerful mechanism for control of the medical profession. The prudent obstetrician often sees no alternative but to monitor electronically. At the same time, the use of EFM reinforces the public misconception that a physician has the tools to adequately predict the effects of perinatal asphyxia to the degree that he or she may be held legally accountable.

IMPACT OF TECHNOLOGY ASSESSMENT

Although the impact of technology assessment on the use of EFM has not been quantified, it is clear that the initial diffusion of EFM was not affected by technology assessment. By the time the first assessment was published in 1979, nearly half of all deliveries in the United States were monitored electronically. In many academic centers the policy at that time was one of universal monitoring. In most hospitals, at least high-risk pregnancies were monitored electronically. The key data in assessing the effectiveness of this technology have come from RCTs. As noted previously, by 1987 nine RCTs had been conducted, but the impact of their results on clinical practice has been limited.

I cannot therefore estimate the impact on EFM of either the increasingly available data on efficacy and safety or formal technology assessment. There is little information, in fact, on the impact of the technology assessment process. The rapid implementation and discontinuation of the Swine Influenza Immunization Program illustrate the dramatic impact that social and political forces can have on the use of technologies.[42] Historically, however, technologies tend to diffuse and disappear slowly, unless there are dramatic circumstances that force an action. The Methods and Evaluation Panels of the Council on Health Care Technology of the Institute of Medicine intend to examine evidence measuring the effectiveness of the technology assessment process.

INFLUENCE OF MEDICAL MALPRACTICE ON THE USE OF ELECTRONIC FETAL MONITORING

There is no doubt that many obstetricians have been encouraged to use EFM because of a fear of liability for not using the "customary procedure." The precise impact of malpractice concerns on the diffusion of EFM, however, has not been measured. More important, this fear of liability may not be well grounded. Careful reading of the relevant legal literature indicates that failure to use EFM should not result in liability, whereas using EFM in a routine labor and delivery may result in malpractice allegations.[43, 44]

The critical legal assumptions regarding liability for not using a procedure are that (a) the procedure provides accurate and reliable information; (b) the information is of value for diagnosis; (c) the effective intervention is feasible following diagnosis; and (d) the procedure is better than other alternatives, in terms not only of effectiveness but also of safety. As noted, however, there is no consensus on these assumptions for EFM. As a result, physicians may not be liable for failing to use EFM, and those who do use EFM may be liable for failing to "keep abreast" or to "use best judgment," or even for "negligence."

In medical malpractice the plaintiff must prove that an injury is the result of the physician's failure to act with "reasonable care." To establish causation, the use (or nonuse) of a technology or procedure must be shown to be the proximate cause of the injury; that is, nonuse (or use) is likely to reduce the risk of injury. If the allegation is that EFM should have been used, it must be shown that the use of EFM would have reduced the risk of injury. If, on the other hand, the allegation is that auscultation, not EFM, should have been used, it must be shown that

EFM use significantly contributed to injury. Under the ordinary standards of negligence, as opposed to negligence standards applied to the medical profession, liability is found more often for using EFM, a monitoring procedure that entails greater risk than auscultation. Even under medical negligence standards, the physician needs only to show that the monitoring technique used (whether EFM or auscultation) adhered to customary practice.

The standards for "reasonable care" in medical liability are often associated with "customary practice." Does the physician possess and employ knowledge and skills in a reasonable manner, comparable to his or her peers? The legal interpretation of liability, however, is not limited to customary practice. In "ordinary negligence," failure to use a safe procedure could entail an inexcusable risk, beyond general standards of reasonableness. A whole industry (or specialty) may be found negligent for failing to adopt a new or safer technology or for prematurely using a new technology. Examples of premature diffusion of technologies in perinatal medicine include the use of high concentrations of oxygen in premature infants (leading to retrolental fibroplasia);[45] prescribing diethylstilbestrol (DES) for pregnant women to prevent miscarriages (leading to vaginal cancer in the children);[46] and prescribing a Dalkon shield, an intrauterine birth control device that was associated with septic spontaneous abortions and pelvic inflammatory disease.[47] Legal decisions in these cases were often based on the physician's duty to keep abreast of scientific knowledge and use the "best judgment" based on that knowledge. Failure to do what a physician knows should be done can result in liability for an unfavorable outcome or injury.

In the case of EFM, because there is no consensus on the efficacy of the procedure and because there are risks (such as cesarean delivery) and costs associated with the practice, there appears to be no universally accepted standard of customary practice. Hence, the use of EFM in a particular case may not be justified.

The law recognizes a wide scope of discretion in the medical profession, and in a situation in which a "reputable minority" favors a particular practice, such as intermittent auscultation, no liability may be found when a physician fails to use a procedure favored by the majority (that is, customary practice). Use of EFM, on the other hand, may not protect the physician against liability in a suit brought because of complications arising from cesarean delivery when the use of an acceptable alternative (intermittent auscultation) was not likely to have led to a cesarean delivery.

The determination of liability will vary with the jurisdiction. "The legal standards employed to determine liability by courts in every jurisdiction do not provide a simple prescription for avoiding malpractice liability. Instead, physicians are required to use sound and reasonable judgment under the circumstances."[48]

What I have described here is how the law is intended to work. In practice, however, decisions are often based on perceptions, both of plaintiffs and defendants. When a child is left with a serious disability, for example, it is difficult not to try to compensate the family and, as a result, find fault with the physician, even if the scientific evidence does not show negligence or incompetence. It is not surprising, therefore, that a 1987 survey conducted by the American College of Obstetricians and Gynecologists of about 2,000 of its members found that most claims are settled out of court.[49] Although EFM was not the focus of the survey, there were a few related findings. First, brain damage of the infant was significantly more likely to be the primary allegation in an obstetrical claim (31 percent) than any other category of primary allegation. In obstetrical claims the use of EFM was present to a significantly higher degree (46 percent) than any other characteristic. No specific details were provided on EFM-related litigation.

Given these circumstances, what can the obstetrician do to protect against malpractice claims? From the legal perspective, the best protection is informed consent.[50] A person has the legal right to make informed choices, and a well-informed patient is less likely to sue a physician. Moreover, because no technology or procedure can guarantee a perfect outcome, informing a patient will help to avoid unrealistic expectations. There is, of course, the difficulty of providing the patient with complete and unbiased information. A 1975 study of obstetrical and gynecological malpractice verdicts found that the "medical consumer frequently looks back upon this [the informed consent process] as 'selling the procedure' rather than giving information and getting consent."[51] It is incumbent on the physician, therefore, to conscientiously provide a thorough, clear presentation of a procedure, including both the benefits and the risks. This practice will not only foster better physician-patient interaction but will serve the physician well in the event that mother and child suffer an injury or other adverse outcome.

Electronic fetal monitoring was introduced at a time when the obstetrician's primary concern was shifting from the mother to the fetus and newborn child. The 1970s were also a time of increasing use of technology in obstetrics and other areas of medicine. The obstetrician, motivated by a desire to protect the unborn child, was offered a variety of new tools—all promising not only to deliver more information but also to improve the outcomes of labor and delivery. As a consequence, EFM diffused rapidly, and its use has become standard medical practice throughout the United States. Unlike most technologies, EFM underwent a formal technology assessment—but only after it had become a standard practice. The impact of technology assessment and medical malpractice on the diffusion of EFM is not clear, but it was probably minor compared with the impact of the other factors governing diffusion. Practicing defensive medicine because of the fear of litigation may have a greater impact on the continued use of EFM in clinical practice.

It is interesting to note that the obstetrical community continues to debate the appropriate use of EFM. In April 1988 a committee of the American College of Obstetricians and Gynecologists recommended that the college endorse the position that EFM remains a useful tool but that even in high-risk pregnancies monitoring by auscultation is acceptable clinical practice.[52]

REFERENCES

1. Banta, H. D., and S. B. Thacker. 1979. Costs and Benefits of Electronic Fetal Monitoring: A Review of the Literature. DHEW Pub. no. (PHS) 79-3245. Hyattsville, Md.: National Center for Health Services Research.
2. Hon, E. H., and O. W. Hess. 1957. Instrumentation of fetal electrocardiography. Science 125:553–554.
3. Hon, E. H. 1959. The fetal heart rate patterns preceding death in uterus. Am. J. Obstet. Gynecol. 78:47–56.
4. Hon, E. H. 1960. Apparatus for continuous monitoring of the fetal heart rate. Yale J. Biol. Med. 32:397–399.
5. Hehre, F. W. 1974. Biophysical monitoring by fetal electrocardiography. Clin. Anesth. 10:81–101.
6. Hon, E. H., R. H. Paul, and R. W. Hon. 1972. Electronic evaluation of FHR. XI. Description of a spiral electrode. Obstet. Gynecol. 40:362–365.
7. Hehre. 1974; see note 5.
8. Saling, E. 1961. Neue Untersuch Ungsmoglichkeiten des Kindes Unter Geburt (Einfuhrung and Grundlagen). Zent. Gynäkol. 83:1906–1908.
9. Dilts, P. V. 1976. Current practices in antepartum and intrapartum fetal monitoring. Am. J. Obstet. Gynecol. 126:491–494.
10. Paul, R. H., and E. H. Hon. 1970. A clinical fetal monitor. Obstet. Gynecol. 35:161–169.
11. Heldford, A. J., C. N. Walker, and M. E. Wade. 1976. Do we need fetal monitoring in a community hospital? Trans. Pac. Coast Obstet. Gynecol. Soc. 43:25–30.
12. Lee, W. K., and M. S. Baggish. 1976. The effect of unselected intrapartum fetal monitoring. Obstet. Gynecol. 47:516–520.
13. Zdeb, M. S., and V. M. Logrillo. 1979. Prenatal monitoring in upstate New York. Am. J. Public Health 69:499–501.
14. Placek, P. J., K. G. Keppel, S. M. Taffel, and T. L. Liss. 1984. Electronic fetal monitoring in relation to cesarean section delivery for live births and still births in the U.S. Public Health Rep. 99:173–183.
15. Banta, H. D., and S. B. Thacker. 1979. Assessing the costs and benefits of electronic fetal monitoring. Obstet. Gynecol. Survey 34:627–642.
16. Thacker, S. B. 1987. The efficacy of intrapartum electronic fetal monitoring. Am. J. Obstet. Gynecol. 156:24–30.

17. Shy, K. K., E. B. Larson, and D. A. Luthy. 1987. Evaluating a new technology: The effectiveness of electronic fetal heart rate monitoring. Ann. Rev. Public Health 8:165–190.
18. Banta, H. D., C. J. Behney, and J. S. Willems. 1981. Toward Rational Technology in Medicine. New York: Springer.
19. Renou, P., A. Chang, I. Anderson, and C. Wood. 1976. Interpretation of the continuous fetal heart rate monitor. Obstet. Gynecol. 126:470–476.
20. Haverkamp, A. D., M. Orleans, S. Langendoerfer, J. McFee, J. Murphy, and H. E. Thompson. 1979. A controlled trial of the differential effects of intrapartum fetal monitoring. Am. J. Obstet. Gynecol. 134:399–412.
21. MacDonald, D., A. Grant, M. Sheridan-Pereira, P. Boylan, and I. Chalmers. 1985. The Dublin randomized controlled trial of intrapartum fetal heart rate monitoring. Am. J. Obstet. Gynecol. 152:524–539.
22. Renou et al. 1976; see note 19.
23. Wood, C., P. Renou, J. Oates, E. Farrel, N. Beischer, and I. Anderson. 1981. A controlled trial of fetal heart rate monitoring in a low-risk obstetric population. Am. J. Obstet. Gynecol. 141:527–534.
24. Haverkamp et al. 1979; see note 20.
25. Neldman, S., M. Oster, P. K. Hansen, J. Nim, S. F. Smith, and J. Hertel. 1986. Intrapartum fetal heart rate monitoring in a combined low- and high-risk population: A controlled clinical trial. Eur. J. Obstet. Gynecol. Reprod. Biol. 12:1–11.
26. MacDonald et al. 1985; see note 21.
27. Haverkamp, A. D., H. E. Thompson, J. G. McFee, and C. Cetrulo. 1976. The evaluation of continuous fetal heart rate monitoring in high-risk pregnancy. Am. J. Obstet. Gynecol. 125:310–317.
28. Kelso, I. M., R. J. Parsons, G. F. Lawrence, S. S. Arora, D. K. Edmonds, and I. D. Cooke. 1978. An assessment of continuous fetal heart rate monitoring in labor. Am. J. Obstet. Gynecol. 131:526–532.
29. Leveno, K. S., F. G. Cunningham, S. Nelson, M. Roark, M. L. Williams, D. Guzick, S. Dowling, C. R. Rosenfeld, and A. Buckley. 1986. A prospective comparison of selective and universal electronic fetal monitoring in 34,995 pregnancies. N. Eng. J. Med. 315:615–619.
30. MacDonald et al. 1985; see note 21.
31. Leveno et al. 1986; see note 29.
32. Luthy, D. A., K. K. Shy, G. Van Bell, E. B. Larson, J. P. Hughes, T. J. Benedetti, Z. A. Brown, S. Effer, J. F. King, and M. A. Stenchever. 1987. A randomized trial of electronic fetal monitoring in premature labor. Obstet. Gynecol. 69:687–695.
33. Fineberg, H. F. 1985. Effects of clinical evaluation on the diffusion of medical technology. Pp. 176–210 in Assessing Medical Technologies. Washington, D.C.: National Academy Press.
34. Banta, H. D., and S. B. Thacker. 1979. Policies toward medical technology: The case of electronic fetal monitoring. Am. J. Public Health 69:931–935.
35. Haverkamp et al. 1979; see note 20.
36. Haverkamp et al. 1976; see note 27.
37. National Institute of Child Health and Human Development. 1979. Part III: Predictors of Fetal Distress. I. Antenatal Diagnosis. NIH Pub. no. 79-1973:1–199. Washington, D.C.: Government Printing Office.
38. Kosecoff, J., D. E. Kanouse, W. H. Rogers, L. McCloskey, C. M. Winslow, and R. H. Brook. 1987. Effects of the National Institutes of Health Consensus Development Conference on physician practice. JAMA 258:2708–2713.

39. Pub. L. No. 94-295.
40. Anderson, C. G. 1975. Monitoring in labor, a patient cost survey. Contemp. Obstet. Gynecol. 6:102–104.
41. Dans, P. E., J. P. Weiner, and S. E. Otter. 1985. Peer Review Organizations: Promises and potential pitfalls. N. Eng. J. Med. 313:1131–1137.
42. Neustadt, R. E., and H. V. Fineberg. 1978. The Swine Flu Affair: Decision-making on a Slippery Disease. Washington, D.C.: U.S. Department of Health, Education, and Welfare.
43. Gilfix, M. G. 1984. Electronic fetal monitoring: Physician liability and informed consent. Am. J. Law Med. 10:31–90.
44. Katz, B. F. 1979. Electronic fetal monitoring and the law. Birth Fam. J. 6:251–258.
45. Silverman, W. 1980. Retrolental Fibroplasia: A Modern Parable. Orlando, Fla.: Grune and Stratton.
46. Gunning, J. E. 1976. The DES story. Obstet. Gynecol. Survey 31:827–833.
47. Layde, P. M. 1983. Pelvic inflammatory disease and the Dalkon shield. JAMA 250:796–797.
48. Gilfix. 1984; see note 43.
49. American College of Obstetricians and Gynecologists. 1988. Professional Liability and Its Effects: Report of a 1987 Survey of ACOG's Membership. Washington, D.C.
50. Gilfix. 1984; see note 43.
51. Shearer, M., M. Raphael, and M. Cattani. 1976. A survey of California OB-GYN malpractice verdicts in 1974 with recommendations for expediting informed consent. Birth Fam. J. 3:59, 64.
52. Cogen, J. 1988. ACOG considers new guidelines for monitoring and labor. Ob/Gyn News 23:1, 43.

Is the Rising Rate of Cesarean Sections a Result of More Defensive Medicine?

BENJAMIN P. SACHS, M.D., M.P.H.

In the United States today, almost 1 in 4 infants is delivered by cesarean section. The marked rise in the rate of use of this procedure over the last decade has coincided with a changing medical-legal environment. In this chapter I address the question of whether there is a relationship between the medical-legal climate and the rising rate of cesarean sections. To address this difficult question, I review the epidemiology of cesarean sections, discuss the causes for the rise in the rate, and examine the possible relationship of that rise to the practice of defensive medicine.

HISTORICAL PERSPECTIVE

Cesarean deliveries were rarely performed in the United States and Europe prior to the end of the nineteenth century.[1] The first reported cesarean section by a physician in the United States was performed in 1827 by John Lambert Richmond.[2] Initially, cesarean sections resulted in high maternal morbidity and mortality because surgeons believed that the uterus should be left unsutured. American physicians—in particular, Frank E. Polin, from Springfield, Kentucky—were at the forefront of demonstrating the importance of suturing the uterus following a cesarean delivery.[3] In 1868 Brickell published the first American report of the use of sutures.[4]

The safety of the surgery was further improved by the recognition that timeliness was important. Harris and Sanger demonstrated that an early cesarean section would improve maternal outcome.[5, 6] The first to recommend a vertical incision through the lower uterine segment was Osiander of Goettingen in 1805.[7] Kara of Heidelberg described a low transverse incision in 1881, and Kronig furthered the work of Kara by recommending a uterovesicle peritoneal reflection.[8]

In 1933 a White House Conference on Child Health and Protection was held.[9] In New York at that time the state maternal mortality committee reported an incidence of cesarean section delivery of 2.2 percent. The maternal loss from cesarean section was reported to range from 4.2 to 16.1 percent, with one-fifth of all maternal deaths occurring among women who underwent a cesarean section. However, this report stressed that the high mortality was due as much to preexisting conditions as to the procedure itself.[10]

EPIDEMIOLOGY OF CESAREAN SECTIONS

There has been a dramatic rise in the rate of cesarean delivery, from less than 5 percent before 1965 to 24.1 percent in 1986.[11] The primary cesarean section rate appears to be leveling off at 17.4 percent, having risen from 4.2 percent in 1970.[12] If the current rate of increase continues, by the year 2000 the total cesarean section rate will be 40 percent; for women aged 35 years and older, it may reach 50 percent.[13]

A National Institutes of Health (NIH) task force examined the reasons for the increase in the cesarean section rate between 1970 and 1978 (Table 1).[14] It reported that 30 percent of the rise was due to a diagnosis of dystocia, 25 to 30 percent to repeat cesarean sections, 10 to 25 percent to breech presentation, and 10 to 15 percent to fetal distress. The further rise that occurred between 1980 and 1985 was recently examined, with the following findings: 48 percent of the increase was due to a previous cesarean section, 5 percent to breech infants, 29 percent to dystocia, 16 percent to fetal distress, and 2 percent to other factors.[15] The major difference between the two analyses is a lower incidence of breech infants and a higher incidence of repeat cesarean sections in the later analysis.

Demographic Factors

A number of demographic factors influence the frequency of cesarean section deliveries. These include the following.

Maternal Age

Women aged 30 years and older have a two- to threefold higher cesarean section rate.[16, 17] The reason is unclear, but it has been sug-

TABLE 1 Contribution of Major Indications to the Increase in Rates of Cesarean Section, 1970–1978 and 1980–1985

	Contribution to Increase (%)	
Indication	1970–1978[a]	1980–1985[b]
Increase in rate[c]	6–15	18–24
Repeat cesarean section	25–30	48
Dystocia	30	29
Fetal distress	10–15	16
Breech	10–25	5
Other	0–25	2

[a]NIH Consensus Development Task Force. 1981. Statement on cesarean childbirth. Am. J. Obstet. Gynecol. 139:902–909.

[b]Taffel, S. M., P. J. Placek, and T. Liss. 1987. Trends in the United States cesarean section rate and reasons for the 1980–85 rise. Am. J. Public Health 77:955–59.

[c]Number of cesarean sections, primary plus repeat, per 100 deliveries; rounded figures.

gested that it is due to a higher incidence of dysfunctional labor and therefore more sedation. As more women delay childbirth, the issue of the high cesarean section rate for the older first-time mother becomes more significant.

Prenatal Care

There is no clear relationship between the presence or absence of prenatal care and the cesarean section rate.[18] In any such analysis there are many confounding variables, such as socioeconomic factors, race, parity, and so on.

Maternal Demographics

Maternal demographics include marital status, education, and ethnic background. Again, it is unclear from the literature whether these factors affect the rate of cesarean delivery.[19, 20]

Hospital Teaching Status

Teaching hospitals are often large facilities that are set in cities and that serve high-risk populations. Furthermore, they often have special-care nurseries. Logically, teaching hospitals should have higher cesarean section rates than other hospitals; a 1981 Massachusetts study, however, found that the cesarean section rate for first births varied only from 0 to 31.4 percent, with an average of 18.5 percent.[21]

Only 1 of the 10 hospitals with the highest rates had a neonatal intensive care unit.

Private or Clinic Care

In four Brooklyn hospitals that accounted for 65,647 deliveries between 1977 and 1982, it was found that private physicians performed significantly more cesarean sections than house officers and attending physicians.[22] Diagnoses of dystocia, malpresentation, or fetal distress were more likely to be made by private physicians. Private patients' infants had lower mortality rates, but they also had a significantly higher incidence of low Apgar scores and birth injuries than the infants of clinic patients.

Hospital Ownership

There is no clear relationship between hospital ownership and the cesarean delivery rate.[23] If there were, then the often-cited economic incentives could be held responsible for the high cesarean section rate. In an analysis of data from hospitals in 1981 Placek and colleagues showed that the highest cesarean section rates were in proprietary hospitals, followed by nonprofit hospitals, and then government hospitals.[24] In contrast, a New York City study found nonprofit hospitals and proprietary hospitals to have similar rates.[25]

Insurance Coverage

A recent study showed higher cesarean section rates for patients with Blue Cross-Blue Shield or other private insurance.[26] The lowest rates were seen in self-paying patients and Medicaid patients. These findings were true both in 1980 and 1986.

Comparison of National Cesarean Section Rates

There has been a marked rise in the frequency of cesarean deliveries in Europe and in Australia and New Zealand (Table 2), but the highest rates are found in the United States.[27] National differences are related to differences in obstetrical practice with regard to complications in pregnancy and delivery and the frequency of vaginal deliveries following a cesarean section. The practice of repeat cesarean sections was undoubtedly a major contributor to the higher rate in the United States. Also of interest is the higher incidence of the diagnosis of fetal distress in the United States, compared with the other countries.

TABLE **2** Cesarean Section Rates (as percentage) in Selected Countries, 1970–1973 and 1981–1983

Country	1970–1973	1981–1983	Diagnosis of Fetal Distress (% of all deliveries)
Australia	4	14	—
Denmark	6	13	22
Hungary	6	10	27
New Zealand	4	10	29
England and Wales	5	10	35
United States	6	20	69

SOURCE: Adapted from Notzon, F. C., P. J. Placek, and S. M. Taffel. 1987. Comparisons of national cesarian-section rates. N. Eng. J. Med. 316:386–389.

ELECTRONIC FETAL MONITORING

The technical ability to monitor the fetus continuously during birth was developed in the 1960s. Originally intended for the management of high-risk obstetrical cases, electronic fetal monitoring (EFM) has become almost routine for deliveries in the United States—despite a number of recent reports that routine fetal monitoring does not improve the outcome in low-risk obstetrical patients.[28, 29] The widespread use of EFM has lead to a marked increase in the cesarean section rate, for a number of reasons.

1. The predictive value of electronic fetal monitoring is poor.[30] With increased use of EFM for low-risk patients, the predictive value will be even lower, resulting in an increased cesarean section rate.

2. A method of further evaluating the pattern of the fetal heart rate is to measure the pH of blood samples from the fetus's scalp. However, this procedure is available only in a minority of obstetrical services in the United States.

3. In the current medical-legal environment, in my opinion, fetal heart rate tracings are likely to be overread, leading to more cesarean deliveries.

4. The objective of fetal monitoring is to detect a fetus that is in distress, with the objective of performing either a forceps or a cesarean delivery. Thus, fetal monitoring by itself will increase the rate of intervention.

5. Although difficult to prove, it is thought that there is a higher incidence of dystocia among women who have continuous electronic fetal monitoring, the reason being that they are unable to walk. They are therefore less able to tolerate labor and require more sedation.

DYSTOCIA

Dystocia is a catchall phrase that includes failure to progress in labor and cephalopelvic disproportion. There has not been a marked rise in the birthweight of U.S. infants between 1980 and 1985; therefore, a change in clinical practice must have caused the rise in this diagnosis, which led to a 29 percent increase in cesarean deliveries during this period.[31] This area has not been thoroughly studied; from personal experience, however, I would judge that because of the current medical-legal climate, there has been a decrease in midforceps deliveries. The other explanation may be the widespread use of fetal monitoring and its relationship to dystocia, as discussed earlier.

BREECH PRESENTATION

Between 1980 and 1985, 5 percent of the increase in the cesarean section rate was related to breech presentations.[32] The incidence of an infant presenting by the breech at term is approximately 3 percent. Most clinical studies have shown that certain types of breech infants can safely be delivered vaginally. For others, such as a complete breech or a footling breech, the risk of a vaginal delivery is increased, albeit by a small amount. Despite there being acceptable guidelines for the vaginal delivery of breech infants, in many institutions today all infants who present by the breech are delivered by cesarean section. The question is clearly, why? Again, my impression is that the medical-legal environment is responsible. With so few vaginal breech deliveries, there is less opportunity to educate residents; we have therefore an increasing pool of physicians with little or no experience in performing such deliveries.

REPEAT CESAREAN SECTIONS

Repeat cesarean sections were responsible for 48 percent of the increase in the cesarean section rate between 1980 and 1985.[33] The dictum "once a cesarean section, always a cesarean" was originally put forward by E. B. Cragin, chairman of the Department of Obstetrics and Gynecology at Columbia University College of Physicians and Surgeons at the beginning of the twentieth century.[34] At that time the frequency of uterine rupture was higher than it is today because many more patients had had a classical cesarean section. In contrast, most patients today have a low transverse incision, which has been shown in many studies to allow for safe vaginal delivery in a subsequent pregnancy.[35] In a review of vaginal deliveries following prior cesarean sections the incidence of uterine rupture was 0.7 percent; the incidence of perinatal death (fetal and infant) was 0.93 per 1,000 births.[36] Two of the three perinatal deaths in this study involved patients who had had a prior classical uterine incision. Of note was the fact that two-thirds of the patients in this series of 4,729 patients cared for in 11 institutions underwent successful trials of labor.

The American College of Obstetricians and Gynecologists (ACOG) has put forward the following guidelines for patients undergoing a trial of labor.[37] Labor is indicated for all patients except those who have repeated contraindications to a vaginal delivery. There should be a single infant presenting by the vertex and weighing not more than 4,000 grams. The mother should have had only one prior low transverse incision, with no extension, and the type of incision should be confirmed by a written operative report. Labor is indicated even for women whose previous cesarean section was for dystocia. Technical support should be available in hospital, including skilled nurses, a staff obstetrician, a pediatrician, and an anesthesiologist. Furthermore, an adequate blood bank with compatible blood should be available and staffed 24 hours a day. Electronic fetal monitoring is advisable intrapartum. Finally, there should be immediate access to an operating room.

Given the preponderance of evidence that a trial of labor is safe, why are so many patients undergoing elective, repeat cesarean sections? The reasons might include convenience for both the physician and the patient, although in some cases (e.g., a small community hospital), given the ACOG guidelines, a more substantive reason might be the inability to provide sufficient support for a woman undergoing labor. As described, the risks are very small; nevertheless, in the current medical-legal environment a trial of labor that does not go well and for which the guidelines have not been met would be held against the attending physician and institution. This explanation, I believe, accounts for only a small fraction of the large number of repeat cesarean sections.

RISKS ASSOCIATED WITH CESAREAN SECTION

If the medical-legal environment is driving up the cesarean section rate, is it at the expense of the mother? The maternal mortality rate is defined as the number of maternal deaths during pregnancy and within a set time postpartum per 100,000 live births.[38] For deaths directly related to the cesarean section, the rate in five American and two European studies ranged from 0 to 60.7 per 100,000 cesarean sections.[39, 40] The mean was 27 deaths per 100,000 cesarean sections (with a 95 percent confidence limit, ± 15.1). It is difficult to compare these seven studies as two were hospital based, three were statewide reviews, and two dealt with national statistics. Nevertheless, from these data it would appear that the risk of cesarean section did differ by country and, in the United States, by region.

A more recent study, carried out under the aegis of the Committee on Maternal Welfare of the Commonwealth of Massachusetts, found that between 1954 and 1985 there were 886 maternal deaths in Massachusetts.[41] The maternal mortality rate fell from 50 deaths per 100,000 live births (1954–1957) to 10 (1982–1985). During this same time the cesarean section rate rose dramatically, from 13.9 percent in 1976 to 21.8 percent in 1984. There were 121,217 cesarean sections with 27 deaths, giving a mortality rate of 22.2 per 100,000 cesarean sections. However, only 7 of these deaths were directly related to the operative procedure, giving a mortality rate of 5.8.

A number of studies have attempted to examine the relative risks of a cesarean section and a vaginal delivery.[42, 43] These reports, however, compared all cesarean section-related deaths with all other maternal deaths, thus overestimating the risk of a cesarean section. Between 1976 and 1984 in Massachusetts, as noted earlier, maternal mortality directly related to a cesarean section was 5.8 per 100,000 procedures.[44] In contrast, during the same period there were 57 deaths associated with vaginal delivery, excluding ectopic pregnancies, septic abortions, and nonmaternal deaths. This calculates to a rate of 10.8 deaths per 100,000 vaginal deliveries. Thus, one can conclude that, in Massachusetts in the 1980s, a cesarean section is at least as safe as a vaginal delivery for the mother with respect to mortality. It should be stressed, however, that all studies have shown that a cesarean section is a far more morbid procedure for the mother, with morbidity including increased incidence of infection, longer hospitalization, and problems of bonding with the infant, as well as rarer complications, including hysterectomy and bowel trauma.

The relative safety of cesarean sections clearly must play a part in the decision making in individual cases. If the obstetrician is concerned about the risk, albeit a small one, of increased perinatal morbidity and mortality, he or she will resort to a cesarean section earlier because of the reassurance of the relative safety of the procedure.

HAS THE INCREASED RATE OF CESAREAN SECTIONS LOWERED PERINATAL MORTALITY?

Is there a cause-and-effect relationship between the dramatic rise in the number of cesarean sections performed in the United States over the last decade and the simultaneous decline in neonatal mortality? The analysis of a potential relationship is confounded by a number of issues, the major one being the widespread introduction of neonatal intensive care units and improved neonatal care. The National Maternity Hospital in Dublin has reported a similar decline in perinatal mortality, despite a stable cesarean section rate of approximately 5 percent. A recent article comparing the perinatal outcome in patients delivered at Parkland Memorial Hospital in Dallas and at the National Maternity Hospital in Dublin reported that there was a higher rate of perinatal morbidity in Dublin, presumably as a result of the lower cesarean section rate.[45] Yet when this comparison is extended over more years, there is no longer a difference in either perinatal mortality or morbidity, despite cesarean delivery rate at Parkland Memorial Hospital that is six times higher than the rate at the National Maternity Hospital in Dublin. It is of interest to note that in this Dublin hospital almost 20 percent of the patients delivered infants who weighed more than 4,000 grams.

The contrary point of view was put forth by Williams and Chen in a study in California in which they showed that there was a reduction in perinatal mortality in infants weighing less than 2,000 grams as a result of the advent of neonatal intensive care units and an increase in the cesarean delivery rate.[46] I examined the effects of cesarean section on neonatal mortality rates for breech and low-birthweight vertex infants in Georgia between 1974 and 1978.[47] For 229,241 singleton deliveries, cesarean section improved the neonatal outcome for breech infants and high-risk low-birthweight infants presenting by the vertex.

COST OF CESAREAN SECTIONS

In 1984 health care costs represented 10.6 percent of the gross national product (GNP), with an expenditure of $387 billion. Health care costs are projected to approach 12 percent of the GNP by 1990, with expenditures of $660 billion. If we continue in this fashion, we can expect an expenditure of $1.9 trillion, representing 14 percent of the GNP, by the year 2000. In terms of percentage of GNP, the United States has the most expensive health care system in the world, but statistics for maternal and child health do not reflect this large expenditure. The United States has one of the highest infant mortality rates of all developed countries, with a large disparity in the rates among socioeconomic groups. The high infant mortality rate is largely secondary to a high incidence of prematurity, the rate of which has not changed in almost 20 years.

A cesarean section may improve the outcome for some premature infants but clearly does not affect the number of premature births. The very high cesarean delivery rate in the United States, driven by the medical-legal environment, adds considerably to the cost of health care;

yet the recent rise in the rate has not been shown to have improved the outcome for either mother or infant. The difference in cost between an uncomplicated cesarean section and an uncomplicated vaginal delivery in Boston in 1988 was $4,000–$5,000. This figure assumes a global fee for obstetrical care; thus, the differential will be higher in instances in which the physicians bill for a cesarean versus a vaginal delivery. Furthermore, this figure will clearly vary from hospital to hospital and state to state; nevertheless, it emphasizes the importance of the fiscal issue. If the cesarean section rate could be reduced by 5 percent, it would represent a savings of between $700 and $900 million per annum.

HEALTH POLICY

A 1987 survey of practicing obstetricians by the American College of Obstetricians and Gynecologists found that 46 percent were performing routine fetal monitoring, 41 percent reported a change in their clinical practice because of the medical-legal environment, 33 percent cared for fewer or no high-risk patients at all, and 12 percent were no longer practicing obstetrics.[48] The widespread use of routine EFM is a form of defensive medicine: it reflects the perception among many clinicians that fetal monitoring and a timely cesarean section can keep them out of court. There is some truth in this. A study by the Harvard Risk Management Foundation of 75 single claims between 1976 and 1988 found that the frequency of allegations was 24 percent for fetal distress and only 7 percent for improper cesarean sections.[49]

The most prominent cases with the largest settlements or awards revolve around the issues of cerebral palsy and mental retardation. The epidemiological evidence clearly shows that only a small percentage of the cases that result in cerebral palsy or mental retardation, or both, are secondary to intrapartum events and thus affected by fetal monitoring or a cesarean delivery.[50, 51] Cerebral palsy is defined as "a chronic disability characterized by an aberrant control of movement and posture appearing early in life and not a result of recognized progressive disease." The incidence of cerebral palsy is approximately 2 per 1,000 school-age children. The common association is low weight at birth. The lower the birthweight, the higher the risk of cerebral palsy. In full-term infants with cerebral palsy, only 16 percent of the cases in one series were caused by perinatal events.[52] The prevalence of severe mental retardation is 3–4 per 1,000 children of school age, with mild retardation found in 1–3 percent of children of school age. The most common cause of severe mental retardation is genetic, with only about 18 percent of cases the result of perinatal events.[53] In both animal experimentation and epidemiological studies it has been shown that total asphyxia in full-term infants leads to brain damage and in most cases to perinatal death. (Lack of oxygen that is sustained long enough to cause brain damage usually results in myocardial ischemia and renal damage as well.)

In obstetrical malpractice cases it is often alleged that an instance of cerebral palsy, mental retardation, or both was secondary to intrapartum events. The plaintiff alleges failure to perform a timely cesarean section or misinterpretation of the fetal heart rate tracing, or both, resulting in death or brain damage. This medical-legal concentration on the issues of fetal monitoring and cesarean section is the origin, in my opinion, of the perception among clinicians that they need to perform defensive medicine. It is not helped by the fact that interpretation of a fetal monitor tracing is more of an art than a science.[54] The broader issue relating to the etiology of cerebral palsy and mental retardation is often ignored in this environment.

The Children's Defense Fund in Washington, D.C., has reported a decrease in the availability of obstetrical care, in part as a result of the medical-legal environment. Some contend that this is a financial issue, resulting from lower physician reimbursement for Medicaid patients. In Massachusetts, however, the Medicaid reimbursement rates are the same as those of many private insurance carriers, and there is still a shortage of obstetricians for Medicaid patients. Again, I think that this is fallout from the medical-legal environment, the perception among obstetricians being that Medicaid patients are at higher risk and more likely to sue. This perception may be related in part to the relationship between the physician and the patient: an unexpected bad outcome is more likely to result in a suit if the patient and physician have a poor relationship or no relationship at all. This situation is more frequently the case for Medicaid patients and patients with no insurance.

SUMMARY

There is overwhelming evidence that part of the recent rise in the cesarean section rate in this country is the result of the medical-legal environment. Given the current siege mentality among clinicians, one wonders why the cesarean section rate is not higher. Arguments that the rise in the cesarean section rate is a result of defensive medicine include

1. the widespread use of fetal monitoring (because of the medical-legal environment, fetal monitoring is widely used, even though its poor predictive value for detecting perinatal asphyxia in low-risk patients results in more cesarean sections);[55]
2. the lower incidence of midforceps deliveries;[56]
3. abandonment of vaginal breech deliveries;[57] and

4. physicians' perception that the majority of allegations in obstetrics suits involve the issues of fetal monitoring and failure to perform a timely cesarean section.

Arguments that the higher cesarean section rate is not a form of defensive medicine include

1. a rise in the cesarean section rate in countries that do not have the same tort system as the United States;[58] and
2. dystocia and repeat cesarean sections as important reasons for the rise in the cesarean section rate—they are probably only in part a result of the medical-legal environment.[59]

The high cesarean section rate in the United States is a major public health problem, one that is having and will continue to have a major impact on health care delivery. If the $800 million that could be saved by reducing the cesarean section rate by 5 percent were spent instead on prenatal care and preventive programs, dramatic effects on maternal and child health would be seen. This shift, in my opinion, is very unlikely to occur, given the current medical-legal environment, which has resulted in a siege mentality among clinicians. If one also considers that less than 20 cents on the dollar paid for malpractice premiums is given to injured parties, our current tort system is clearly very expensive, inefficient, and, because of its adverse effects on the delivery of maternity care, dangerous.

REFERENCES

1. Speert, H. 1980. Obstetrics and Gynecology in America: A History. Baltimore, Md.: Waverly Press.
2. Richmond, J. L. 1830. History of a successful case of caesarean operation. Western J. Med. Phys. Sci. 3:485–489.
3. Speert. 1980; see note 1.
4. Brickell, D. W. 1868. A successful case of caesarean section. N. Orleans J. Med. 21:454–466.
5. Harris, R. P. 1887. Cattle-horn lacerations of the abdomen and uterus in pregnant women. Am. J. Obstet. 20:673–685.
6. Sanger, M. 1882. Der Kaiserschnitt Bei Uterusfibromen Nebst Vergleichender Methodik der Section Caesarea und der Porro-operation. Leipzig: Engelmann.
7. DeLee, J. V. 1925. An illustrated history of the low or cervical cesarean section. Trans. Am. Gynecol. Soc. 50:90–107.
8. Speert. 1980; see note 1.
9. Plass, E. D. 1933. Forceps and cesarean section. Pp. 215–247 in White House Conference on Child Health and Protection. Fetal, Newborn, and Maternal Mortality and Morbidity. New York: Appleton-Century.

10. Ibid.
11. Placek, P. J., S. M. Taffel, and M. Moien. 1988. 1986 Cesarean section rise; VBAC inch upward. Am. J. Public Health 78(5):562–563.
12. Ibid.
13. Placek, P. J., S. M. Taffel, and T. L. Liss. 1987. The cesarean future. Am. Demog. 9(9):46–47.
14. National Institutes of Health, Consensus Development Task Force. 1981. Statement on cesarean childbirth. Am. J. Obstet. Gynecol. 139:902–909.
15. Taffel, S. M., P. J. Placek, and T. Liss. 1987. Trends in the United States cesarean section rate and reasons for the 1980–85 rise. Am. J. Public Health 77:955–959.
16. Placek et al. 1987; see note 13.
17. National Institutes of Health. 1981; see note 14.
18. Ibid.
19. Williams, R. L., and W. E. Hawes. 1979. Cesarean section, fetal monitoring and perinatal mortality in California. Am. J. Public Health 69:864–870.
20. Placek, P. J. 1978. Type of delivery associated with social, demographic, maternal health, infant health and health insurance factors. In Findings from the 1972 U.S. National Natality Survey, Part II. Proceedings of the Social Statistics Section, 1977. Washington, D.C.: American Statistical Association.
21. Dars, L. K., S. L. Rosen, and M. T. Hannon. 1984. Cesarean Birth in Massachusetts. Boston: Department of Public Health, Commonwealth of Massachusetts.
22. Haynes, D. E., R. Regt, H. Minkoff, J. Feldman, and R. Schwarz. 1986. Relation of private or clinic care to the cesarean birth rate. N. Eng. J. Med. 315:619–624.
23. National Institutes of Health. 1981; see note 14.
24. Placek, P. J., S. M. Taffel, and M. Moien. 1983. Cesarean section delivery rates: United States, 1981. Am. J. Public Health 73:861–862.
25. Williams and Hawes. 1979; see note 19.
26. Placek, P. J. 1988. Data from 1980 and 1986 National Hospital Discharge Surveys. Personal communication.
27. Watson, F. C., P. J. Placek, and S. M. Taffel. 1987. Comparisons of national cesarean section rates. N. Eng. J. Med. 316:386–389.
28. Leveno, K. S., F. G. Cunningham, S. Nelson, M. Roark, M. L. Williams, D. Guzick, S. Dowling, C. R. Rosenfeld, and A. Buckley. 1986. A prospective comparison of selective and universal electronic fetal monitoring in 34,995 pregnancies. N. Eng. J. Med. 315:615–619.
29. MacDonald, D., A. Grant, M. Sheridan-Pereira, P. Boylan, and I. Chalmers. 1985. The Dublin randomized controlled trial of intrapartum fetal heart rate monitoring. Am. J. Obstet. Gynecol. 152:524–539.
30. Leveno et al. 1986; see note 28. MacDonald et al. 1985; see note 29. Banta, H. D., and S. B. Thacker. 1979. Assessing the costs and benefits of electronic fetal monitoring. Obstet. Gynecol. Survey 34:627–642.
31. Taffel et al. 1987; see note 15.
32. Ibid.
33. Ibid.
34. Cragin, E. B. 1916. Conservatism in obstetrics. N. Y. Med. J. 54:1.
35. Riva, H. L., and J. C. Teich. 1961. Vaginal delivery after cesarean section. Am. J. Obstet. Gynecol. 81:501–510.
36. O'Sullivan, M. J., F. Fumia, K. Holsinger, and A. G. W. McLeod. 1981. Vaginal delivery after cesarean section. Clin. Perinatol. 8:131–143.
37. Committee reports guidelines for vaginal delivery. 1982. ACOG Newsletter 26:1.

38. American College of Obstetricians and Gynecologists. 1974. Standards for obstetrics and gynecology services. Washington, D.C.
39. Harris. 1887; see note 5.
40. Beard, R. W., G. M. Gilshie, and C. A. Knight. 1971. The significance of the changes in the continuous fetal heart rate in the first stage of labor. J. Obstet. Gynaecol. Brit. Commonwealth 78:865–881.
41. Sachs, B. P., J. Yeh, D. Acker, S. Driscoll, B. J. Ransil, D. A. J. Brown, and J. F. Jewett. 1987. Cesarean section—related maternal mortality in Massachusetts, 1954–1985. Obstet. Gynecol. 71:385–388.
42. Frigoletto, F. D., K. J. Ryan, and M. Phillippe. 1980. Maternal mortality rate associated with cesarean section: An appraisal. Am. J. Obstet. Gynecol. 36:969–973.
43. Rubin, G. L., H. B. Peterson, R. W. Rochat, B. J. McCarthy, and J. S. Terry. 1981. Maternal death after cesarean section in Georgia. Am. J. Obstet. Gynecol. 39:681–685.
44. Sachs et al. 1987; see note 41.
45. Leveno, K., G. Cunningham, and J. Pritchard. 1985. Cesarean section: An answer to the House of Horne. Am. J. Obstet. Gynecol. 153:838–844.
46. Williams, R. L., and P. Chen. 1982. Identifying the sources of the recent decline in perinatal mortality rates in California. N. Eng. J. Med. 306:207–214.
47. Sachs, B. P., B. J. McCarthy, G. Rubin, A. Burton, J. Terry, and C. W. Tyler. 1983. Cesarean section: Risk and benefits for mother and fetus. JAMA 250:2157–2159.
48. American College of Obstetricians and Gynecologists. 1988. Professional Liability and Its Effects: Report of a 1987 Survey of ACOG's Membership. Washington, D.C.
49. Risk Management Foundation of the Harvard Medical Institutions, Inc. 1986. Forum 7(4):1–8.
50. Holm, V. A. 1982. The causes of cerebral palsy: A contemporary perspective. JAMA 247:1473–1477.
51. Stein, Z. A., and M. N. Susser. 1980. Mental retardation. Pp. 1266–1283 in Public Health and Preventive Medicine, 11th ed., J. Last, P. Sartwell, K. Maxcy, and M. Rosenau, eds. New York: Appleton-Century-Crofts.
52. Holm. 1982; see note 50.
53. Stein and Susser. 1980; see note 51.
54. Cohen, A. B., H. Klapholz, and M. S. Thompson. 1982. Electronic fetal monitoring and clinical practice. A survey of obstetric opinion. Med. Decision Making 2(1):79–95.
55. Bissonnette, J. M. 1975. Relationship between continuous fetal heart rate patterns and Apgar score in the newborn. Brit. J. Obstet. Gynaecol. 82:24–28. Leveno et al. 1986; see note 28. MacDonald et al. 1985; see note 29. Banta and Thacker. 1979; see note 30.
56. Taffel et al. 1987; see note 15.
57. Ibid.
58. Watson et al. 1987; see note 27.
59. Taffel et al. 1987; see note 15.

Medical Professional Liability in Screening for Genetic Disorders and Birth Defects

NEIL A. HOLTZMAN, M.D., M.P.H.

In the spirit of Jacob Marley I am going to present glimpses of screening past (for phenylketonuria, or PKU), screening present (for fetal neural tube defects using maternal serum alpha-fetoprotein—MSAFP), and screening future (for a wide range of disorders using DNA-based tests). Physicians have been held liable for errors in PKU screening, and some will almost certainly be sued for mistakes in MSAFP testing. Despite its elegance, recombinant DNA technology, which is the basis of future screening, does not solve the problems of the past or present; exposure to liability will become greater as the magnitude of screening increases. Although this discussion is restricted to the problems of only one class of technological innovation, my concluding suggestions on how to reduce the chance of liability apply to many other innovations which, like screening, offer the promise of improving health outcomes.

Screening, as I use the term, involves the testing of a healthy population to predict who is at increased risk of manifesting disease in the future or whose offspring are at increased risk. Because the pool of potential recipients of screening tests is very large (for example, all pregnant women or all newborns), the failure to screen even a small proportion could lead to malpractice suits when someone who was not screened manifests the disease. The less common the disease, the less likely are such suits. They have, nevertheless, occurred for PKU (incidence of about 1 in 12,000) and are more likely for neural tube defects (incidence of about 1 in 1,000).

41

TABLE 1   Definition of Terms Used to Assess Screening

Sensitivity—The probability that a person (or his or her offspring) who will manifest the disease will be detected by screening, that is, will have a positive test result.

Specificity—The probability that a person (or his or her offspring) who will not manifest the disease will have a normal (negative) screening test result.

Predictive value of a positive test result—The probability that a person with a positive test result (or his or her offspring) will manifest the disease.

Reliability (measures of test performance)

Precision—Repeated determinations yield the same result.

Accuracy—The determinations center around the true value.

When screening is legally mandated (as is the case for PKU in most states), when physicians are legally required to *offer* it (as providers of obstetric care must do for MSAFP testing in California), when it becomes the standard of care, or simply when reasonable people think screening should be done (and the capability to perform it is present), providers who fail to screen or offer screening will have a difficult time defending themselves from liability suits.

The failure to screen is only the first problem. Some people destined to manifest a disease will be missed by a test because it is not perfectly sensitive (see Table 1 for definitions). Here, too, the less frequently the disease occurs, the less likely it is that many people will be missed by screening (false negatives). The low frequency of a disorder will not, however, reduce the chance that people who are falsely labeled at risk will bring suit for being needlessly exposed to potentially harmful interventions. When tests for different disorders but with the same sensitivity and specificity are compared, the one for the least common disease will have the greatest chance of being falsely positive. The predictive value of a positive test result depends not only on specificity and sensitivity but on the incidence of the disorder being tested.

It may be easier to defend oneself against liability arising out of false negatives or false positives than against liability arising out of failure to screen at all. This is because the test may be biologically incapable of correctly labeling everyone who is screened. Although the mean concentrations of substances such as phenylalanine or alpha-fetoprotein in maternal blood will be significantly different in those with and those without the respective disorder, considerable variation around the mean will result in some overlap between the two groups. Tests based on qualitative characteristics, such as mutations, may not be foolproof either. A mutation that is known to cause a disease in some people will not cause it in others. One of the difficulties in any individual case in which a mistake has been made is knowing whether it resulted from biological variation (in which case those responsible for the performance of the test would be exonerated) or from faulty performance of the test. Frequently, by the time an error in screening is suspected, the specimen is no longer available for repeat testing. An indirect gauge of the chance that the laboratory made a mistake can be obtained by measuring the reliability of the laboratory on other specimens. When this assessment is done systematically, it is known as proficiency testing.

SCREENING PAST: PHENYLKETONURIA

Phenylketonuria (PKU) is an inherited disorder of amino acid metabolism in which the accumulation of phenylalanine is almost invariably associated with severe mental retardation. In 1954 Bickel and colleagues demonstrated that the concentration of phenylalanine in the blood could be reduced by providing phenylketonurics with diets from which the phenylalanine had been largely removed.[1] The older infants and children in whom the diet was first tried failed to show any persistent, significant reversal of mental retardation, despite the decline in the concentration of the amino acid.[2]

The question remained whether administration of the special diet during or soon after the neonatal period could prevent retardation from appearing in infants with an inherited defect of phenylalanine metabolism. The approach seemed plausible because the placental circulation keeps the PKU fetus's concentration of phenylalanine at or close to normal in utero. We have since learned that early administration of the special diet can prevent retardation in the vast majority of children with PKU.[3] In a few children who have different inherited causes for the increase of phenylalanine in their blood, the low-phenylalanine diet by itself is not effective.[4]

The proportion of infants detected by neonatal testing in whom developmental delay would not be prevented by the low-phenylalanine diet was unknown when in 1965 most states passed laws that required the screening of all newborns for PKU. The laws were passed on the heels of a report by Guthrie and Susi of a simple, inexpensive test for detecting increases of phenylalanine concentrations in the blood.[5] The test required only a few drops of blood, which could be collected on filter paper from a prick in the heel of the newborn, and was therefore applicable to screening. Unfortunately, neither the effectiveness of the low-phenylalanine diet, nor the sensitivity and specificity of the screening test, nor the reliability of the laboratories performing it was established before newborns were routinely screened and those with positive results started on treatment.[6, 7] Without knowledge of the imperfections of the new technology, the probability of unfavorable outcomes and, consequently, of malpractice suits increased.

Problems did materialize. It soon became evident that the phenylalanine concentration that was being used as a criterion for diagnosing PKU was too low. The concentration must be at least five times the upper limit of normal before it is associated with retardation. Some children with lower abnormal concentrations were erroneously treated and suffered serious protein deficiencies as a result.[8] (Phenylalanine is an essential amino acid; even phenylketonurics require it, although in much smaller amounts than do children without the condition.) Other children were treated before anyone realized that their elevations of phenylalanine were only transient.

The problem of false negatives did not emerge quickly. The developmental delay produced by PKU often does not become evident until the second year of life. Even when examining 2-year-olds with developmental delay, physicians are often slow to attribute the retardation to PKU because they place too much confidence in the validity of the screening test. In 1969 a resident at Johns Hopkins discovered that a 14-month-old infant who had been referred with developmental delay had phenylketonuria. The infant had been screened as a newborn, and the results had been reported as normal. This event, together with the finding that more boys with PKU were being detected by newborn screening than were girls—despite the fact that the genetics of the disorder suggested that equal numbers should be detected—prompted me and my colleagues at Hopkins to conduct a survey of PKU clinics and state health departments.[9] We discovered 23 false negatives and found that the probability of PKU infants being missed was greater the earlier they were screened, particularly for girls. Further confirmation that age of screening was important came from comparing the sensitivity of screening in the United States, where most infants were screened at or before 4 days of age, to that in the United Kingdom, where most infants were screened (in their homes by health visitors) between 6 and 10 days. The sensitivity in the United Kingdom was 100 percent, compared with 93 percent in the United States.[10] These findings suggested a biological basis for the less-than-perfect sensitivity of the screening test in the United States. (Since this study, milk feeding of newborns has started earlier; this practice has been associated with a lower probability of false negatives in early screening in the United States.)

We also found evidence that U.S. screening laboratories differed markedly in the frequency with which they found elevated phenylalanine concentrations, a result that suggested variable quality.[11] On average, there were about 10 false positives for every PKU infant detected. At about the same time, a report from the Centers for Disease Control (CDC) revealed the poor proficiency of several of the laboratories that were routinely performing screening tests.[12] Exacerbating the problem of quality, and making it difficult to control, was the large number of laboratories performing newborn screening tests in the United States.[13] In the United Kingdom and Ireland, where screening programs are centralized and where the communication of results follows well-defined policies, not only was the sensitivity of the PKU test higher than in the United States but the interval between screening and follow-up was much shorter.[14] It became clear that, in view of the chance of test error, as well as the chance of biological false positives, any positive screening test result should be followed up with another determination of blood phenylalanine before diagnosing PKU or beginning treatment. (Follow-up is also needed for other disorders for which newborns are now routinely screened.)

A more recent survey of state health departments by investigators at the CDC revealed 43 PKU infants who had been missed by screening, a minimum of 1.4 percent of all PKU infants screened.[15] (Health departments are unlikely to know of all missed cases.) A few of the infants were missed because a specimen never reached the screening laboratory; a few others were missed because a positive test result was never followed up. Such problems might be obviated if parents were better informed about screening. (Because screening in most states does not require parental consent, parents often do not know their infant has been screened until they are told that the test result is positive.) Most of the missed cases were attributed to the laboratory determination, although it was not usually possible to pinpoint the error or to be certain that it did not result from the biological limitations of the test. Laboratories analyzing relatively small numbers of specimens were more likely to miss infants with PKU than were those with greater test volumes, which suggests that quality problems were important. Legal action was taken in 15 of the 26 cases of which the respondents had adequate knowledge. Many of the cases were still pending in 1986 when the survey was reported, but settlements of up to $3 million have been made.

The problems of PKU screening continue. In 1985 the American Bar Foundation examined the problem of legal liability in newborn screening.[16] It concluded that failure of quality control often increased the likelihood of screening errors and, consequently, of legal liability.

SCREENING PRESENT: MSAFP TESTING FOR NEURAL TUBE DEFECTS

Only after Congress passed amendments to the Food, Drug, and Cosmetic Act in 1976 were manufacturers required to demonstrate the safety and effectiveness of diagnostic test materials and other "medical devices" before they could be marketed. Had such a law been on the books in the mid-1960s, PKU screening might have been better validated before it was incorporated into standard neonatal care. (Phenylalanine kits have since been put in a category by the Food and Drug Administration [FDA] that requires them to meet "performance standards." The FDA, however, still has not established the standards.) As the still-unfolding story of MSAFP testing suggests, determination of the effectiveness of a screening test prior to its marketing does not ensure that it will be used appropriately.

Anencephaly, which is not compatible with more than a few days of survival after birth, and open spina bifida, which almost always results in paralysis below the waist and occasionally in hydrocephalus and mental retardation, are the two most common neural tube defects detectable by MSAFP testing. Together they are found in about 1 in 1,000 live births in the United States. Although their occurrence is genetically influenced in at least some cases, more than 95 percent of affected infants are born to families without a previous history of anencephaly or open spina bifida.

The association between elevated concentrations of AFP in the blood of women in the second trimester of pregnancy and open neural tube defects was discovered by Brock and his colleagues in Scotland in 1974.[17] Medical centers serving areas in the United Kingdom in which the frequency of open spina bifida was several times higher than it was in the United States soon began to screen. The principal reason was to offer women carrying fetuses with neural tube defects the opportunity to terminate their pregnancies.

Considerable data on the sensitivity and specificity of MSAFP testing were amassed in the United Kingdom and in a few other European countries by the time the FDA received applications for premarket approval of MSAFP test kits in the United States. By then it was known that, to detect about 70 percent of fetuses with open spina bifida and 90 percent of those with anencephaly, the upper limit of normal MSAFP would have to be set at about the 95th percentile. This means that 50 out of every 1,000 pregnant women who are *not* carrying an affected fetus will have a positive test result. If only 1 in 1,000 is carrying the affected fetus detectable by the test, then there would be 50 false positives for every true positive, giving a predictive value of a positive result of 2 percent.

It might seem that any test that has such a poor predictive value is not worth doing, particularly if the abortion of unaffected fetuses results. One should recall, however, that tests used in populations in which the disorder being sought has a low prevalence will have low predictive values of positive results, even when the tests have high sensitivity and specificity. The specificity of PKU screening is at least 99.9 percent, but the predictive value of a positive result when the incidence of PKU is 1 in

12,000 live births is only 8 percent. When the specificity is relatively low but the prevalence is high—as is the case for serum cholesterol screening for coronary artery disease in healthy middle-aged men—the predictive values will also be low; only about 30 percent in the case of cholesterol screening.[18]

The likelihood of low predictive values of positive screening test results emphasizes the importance of using follow-up tests to confirm or cancel the positive screening test results. Follow-up for MSAFP tests includes a repeat MSAFP determination; amniocentesis, with measurement of the AFP and characterization of the acetylcholinesterase in the amniotic fluid; and ultrasound examination of the spinal region of the fetus. If these studies are properly conducted and interpreted, the chance that an unaffected fetus will be aborted is less than 1 in 200.[19] When such high probabilities can be attained at costs that are low compared with the costs of treating the disorder without early detection, which is the case for both PKU[20] and neural tube defects,[21] screening is economically justified, provided that most people will accept screening and its sequlae.

The problem with MSAFP testing in the United States is that there is no assurance that providers of obstetrical care recognize the need for follow-up studies or will be able to obtain them in a timely fashion. Fewer than half the medical and pediatric residents at Johns Hopkins, as well as practicing physicians taking continuing education courses there, could correctly estimate the predictive value of a test for a disorder that occurred in 1 of 1,000 people when the test was falsely positive in 5 percent of unaffected people.[22] This is the situation with which a physician is confronted when an MSAFP test is reported positive. Most respondents greatly overestimated the predictive value. Among obstetricians who had participated in educational programs on MSAFP testing, only 22 percent knew that the predictive value of a positive result was less than 5 percent, and only 45 percent knew how to proceed when MSAFP test results were positive.[23] (The percentages answering correctly were higher among obstetricians who subsequently adopted MSAFP screening.)

In evaluating premarket approval applications, the FDA does not take into consideration practitioner preparedness to use a test. Frank Young, the commissioner of the FDA, stated recently:

The FDA also cannot decide for practitioners when a test is appropriate, and under what circumstances any particular test should be used. These are judgments that must be made for individual cases. FDA does not have now or should not have a direct regulatory role in the practice of a physician.[24]

This view was not shared by the American College of Obstetricians and Gynecologists (ACOG) and the American Academy of Pediatrics (AAP) when MSAFP test kits were being considered by the FDA in the late 1970s. Fearing the inappropriate use of the tests and attendant malpractice suits, they urged the FDA to restrict the sale of the kits to laboratories that agreed to coordinate the follow-up of positive test results among referring physicians and centers at which additional tests could be reliably performed.[25] The 1976 amendments gave the FDA the authority to do this. Initially, the FDA proposed the restrictions suggested by the ACOG and the AAP, but in 1983 the agency withdrew the proposal and subsequently approved the marketing of MSAFP kits with virtually no restrictions.[26]

The marketing of new medical devices becomes a potent force for their adoption, even when knowledge and capabilities for appropriate use lag behind. Soon after the FDA gave unrestricted premarket approval to MSAFP kits, the ACOG legal department urged obstetricians to advise all of their prenatal patients of the availability of MSAFP testing and to document in each patient's medical record her decision regarding performance of the test. The rationale was to give obstetricians "the best possible defense" when women who were not tested had babies with neural tube defects.[27] Although the ACOG urged obstetricians to learn more about MSAFP screening and follow-up, it failed to recognize that until obstetricians knew more about the procedures, malpractice could arise out of misuse as well as nonuse of the test.

At least one state, California, has regulated MSAFP testing. Patients' fees are paid to the state program, which then contracts on a competitive basis with eight private and health maintenance organization (HMO) laboratories to perform MSAFP testing, using supplies and protocols provided by the health department. (California has a similar arrangement for newborn screening.) The concentration of AFP in the serum specimens is reported to the health department, which determines whether the values are abnormal. The results are mailed to the referring physician, and positive results are also sent by computer to 14 regional genetic centers. The center nearest the patient contacts her physician by telephone and arranges appropriate follow-up.[28] Whether these restrictions will reduce malpractice claims and awards for MSAFP testing remains to be seen. The California system has also facilitated the collection of data on the association between low concentrations of AFP in the mother's blood and the occurrence of Down's syndrome in the fetus.[29]

Our finding that obstetricians who subsequently performed MSAFP testing had better knowledge of screening after participating in rudimentary education programs than those who did not adopt it[30] suggests that physicians who will adopt a new technology are receptive to learning more about it. Unfortunately, the opportunities to do so are not always present. If federal or state agencies were to require such education, the chance of misuse might be reduced. Going one step further, third-party payers could require physicians to demonstrate an understanding of how a new technology should be used before reimbursing them for providing it. Technologies that have the greatest potential for misuse could be singled out for this approach. Third-party payers are more likely to be interested when misuse will increase their costs of providing patient care. These costs do not usually include the costs of malpractice litigation. A more fundamental solution is to teach medical students and house officers to appreciate the dangers and difficulties posed by new technologies, including, in the area of screening, the probabilistic nature of test results.

SCREENING FUTURE: DNA-BASED TESTING

Until the advent of recombinant DNA technology, relatively few genetic disorders or birth defects were amenable to screening. There had to be some substance in a readily accessible body tissue, such as blood, whose quantity or quality indicated increased risk of future disease in the person being tested or in his or her offspring. For many disorders, such substances were unknown; for others, they could not be measured in readily accessible tissues. Recombinant DNA technology removes both of these constraints. Analysis of the DNA of white blood cells of children or adults, or easily accessible chorionic villi or amniotic fluid cells of fetuses, will reveal the presence of disease-causing or susceptibility-conferring genetic variants (alleles) even when the gene is not active at the time of testing or in the tissue used for testing. These variants arose, often several generations earlier, as a result of mutation.

Before such analysis can be used for screening, scientists must identify the disease-causing or susceptibility-conferring allele. This identification can be accomplished with the new technology even when nothing is known about the normal function of the gene. (The following discussion is abridged from reference 31, in which citations can be found.) The first step is to localize the gene responsible for the disease of interest to a specific region of one of the 22 autosomes or the X or Y sex chromosomes. To accomplish this, blood is needed from affected and unaffected individuals in families in which there is strong evidence for Mendelian inheritance of the disease. The genes for several rare disorders have been localized, as have the genes for cystic fibrosis, Duchenne-type muscular dystrophy, adult polycystic disease, familial hypercholesterolemia, some forms of retinoblastoma, Alzheimer's disease, and bipolar affective (manic-depressive) disorder. In the next few years, genes that play a role in breast and lung cancer, hypertension, peripheral vascular disease, peptic ulcer, and schizophrenia are likely to be localized.

Once the gene has been localized, it is possible to predict the risk of future disease in asymptomatic individuals, or in fetuses, who belong to families in which the disease has already occurred on an inherited basis. Localization does not permit population-based screening.

Before screening is possible, the segment of DNA that constitutes the gene of interest must be identified and the DNA of the normal allele of the gene distinguished from the DNA of disease-causing or suscep-tibility-conferring alleles. These activities have already been carried out for Duchenne-type muscular dystrophy, familial hypercholes-terolemia, retinoblastoma, sickle-cell anemia, thalassemia, hemo-philia, and a few rare disorders, including PKU. A DNA sequence that increases the risk of insulin-dependent diabetes mellitus has recently been discovered. Because great strides have been made in simpli-fying the technology, it will not be long before companies that are currently developing DNA-based tests for genetic disorders will be ap-plying to the FDA for premarket approval.[32] Tests may eventually be-come so easy to perform that physicians will use them in their office laboratories.

In discussing screening past and screening present, I stressed the importance of follow-up. For many of the disorders for which DNA-based screening will be developed, follow-up is no less important, but confirm-atory tests, such as those available for PKU or neural tube defects, may not exist.

It is true that DNA-based tests for disorders that are inherited in a straightforward Mendelian fashion (e.g., PKU or sickle-cell anemia) will be more specific than current tests for these disorders because they directly detect disease-causing mutations. Such disorders, however, are not the only ones for which tests are being developed. Searching for larger markets, the biotechnology companies working in this area are very interested in tests for common disorders—cardiovascular disease, cancer, and mental illness.[33] In some families persons possessing alleles capable of causing these diseases will always manifest the disease, but this trend will not be the case in all families. Differences in alleles at other, modifying loci or differences in environmental factors will affect the expressivity of the gene. Until we can determine the presence of these other factors—a task in which success may prove elusive—the predictive value of positive DNA-based tests may not be very high. Furthermore, until we understand more about the early, presymptoma-tic stages of these disorders, tests that confirm or cancel the positive screening test result will not be available.

It should be possible to determine the predictive value of DNA-based screening tests. This determination can be accomplished most quickly by performing the tests on a large number of unrelated people who are past the age at which the disease usually appears. The number of positive tests in people who remain free of symptoms, divided by the total number of positive tests (in those with and without manifestations of the disease), will approximate the predictive value of the test in younger individuals. The approach will also indicate the sensitivity of the test. For many diseases, more than one allele will be capable of causing the disease (an example of genetic heterogeneity). Tests that fail to detect all of these alleles will not be perfectly sensitive. Data on sensitivity, specificity, and predictive value should be required as part of the premarket approval application and should be made known to the health providers using the tests.

Genetic screening in the future will involve not only pregnant women and newborns but children and young adults. Test results that convey the risk of future disease in the person being tested will lead some people to modify their life styles or take medications to lower their risk of future disease. Test results indicating that the person being tested is the carrier of an allele that would place his or her offspring at increased risk will lead some people to avoid the conception or birth of such children. Much remains to be learned about how high risks have to be before people will act to reduce or avoid them and how people's tolerance for risk varies. Health providers also have a lot to learn about how to communicate risks objectively and effectively. Genetic counseling will be an important part of screening in the future, but the number of specially trained counselors is too few to meet the anticipated demand. Even if people do not want to know their own risks, insurance companies and employers will be interested in using genetic screening to identify people at risk for future disease or premature death. Insurance companies will not insure people at increased risk of some costly diseases—at least not at standard premiums—and employers could refuse to hire workers at increased risk to keep their health benefits costs down and reduce the chance of harmful reactions to the work place on the part of susceptible persons.

As new tests are marketed, they will rapidly become the standard of care, as is now happening with MSAFP testing. The fear of liability is not deterring the development of new tests, and it will not deter the adoption of them once they are marketed. In several recent court decisions parents of affected children and the children themselves have been awarded damages because predictive genetic tests were not performed.[34] Providers will test even when they have inadequate understanding of the probabilistic nature of the results and are unable to counsel clients effectively. As DNA-based tests will be both falsely negative (owing to genetic heterogeneity) and falsely positive (owing to diminished expressivity), suits will arise unless there is widespread recognition that the tests cannot give definitive answers. The dangers of liability will be further increased by testing in laboratories whose proficiency has not been demonstrated.

CONCLUSIONS

From testing for one rare disorder 25 years ago, genetic screening has evolved to the point where screening for a wide range of disorders—some of them contributing significantly to total morbidity and mortality—is technically feasible. For those genetic disorders whose manifestations can be prevented, delayed, or ameliorated only by presymptomatic intervention, genetic screening provides a unique opportunity to reduce the magnitude of disability. For genetic disorders for which effective interventions have not been developed, screening can identify individuals or couples at risk of having affected offspring, giving them the option of avoiding conception (and having children through adoption, surrogate motherhood, or ovum, embryo, or sperm donation) or birth (by prenatal diagnosis and abortion). Although not everyone will view these options as benefits, there is little doubt that they will reduce the burden of disease. Yet in doing so there are dangers of misuse. My interest here is with misuse that increases the chance of professional liability and with what can be done to reduce that chance.

The fear of malpractice if they do not screen will prompt many physicians to offer screening. This practice will reduce the number of suits brought because of failure to screen. When screening is offered in institutional settings (e.g., hospitals or HMOs), systems that flag eligible patients who have not been screened could reduce the chance of unintentional failure to screen.

The chance of incurring liability could soon be greater because of misuse of technology than because of nonuse. As very few, if any, population-based tests will be perfectly sensitive and specific, some people will have false-negative results and others false-positive results. Sensitivity and specificity of the test should be determined under screening conditions before tests are approved for marketing. The FDA has the authority to carry out this recommendation.

Once a test is approved, the laboratories performing it should be monitored for proficiency. At present, the system of laboratory regulation is inadequate and varies from state to state. The role of the federal government, established under the Clinical Laboratory Improvement

Act of 1967, has diminished in recent years, although the Health Care Financing Administration performs some inspections. The College of American Pathologists organizes voluntary proficiency testing programs. Because DNA-based tests represent a departure from other types of tests, the ability of laboratories to perform the tests reliably should be specifically examined.

Limiting and centralizing the number of laboratories that will be reimbursed for performing a test—as California has done for newborn and MSAFP screening—will probably improve laboratory quality; it will certainly make it easier to monitor. The trend, however, is toward further decentralization of laboratories. More tests are being performed in physicians' office laboratories; as the technology is simplified, genetic tests could be performed there as well. Very few states regulate physicians' office laboratories.

Health providers must be taught to recognize the probabilistic nature of screening test results. With proper understanding, they would not hesitate to screen again if they encountered a high-risk situation in a person with a negative test result, and they would confirm positive screening test results before taking potentially dangerous or irreversible action. In offering screening and in communicating results, properly trained providers would counsel their patients about the uncertainty attached to screening. This counseling is particularly important when no confirmatory tests are available.

Until curriculum changes ensure that the vast majority of medical school graduates understand how to interpret screening test results, other measures are needed to reduce the chance of misuse and potential liability. Third-party payers should consider requiring some demonstration of competence before they reimburse providers for tests. Alternatively, states could require—as California has done—the involvement of geneticists or other specialists in the follow-up of persons with positive results.

The scope of genetic screening in the future is so large that it is likely to involve most people in making decisions about screening that conflict with their beliefs or attitudes. To prepare people to make these decisions, much more extensive education is needed about human genetics and the implications of genetic testing. As there is no assurance that everyone will either be taught or will learn the issues involved in testing, fully informed consent is essential to preserve individual autonomy and to ensure that the individual understands the reasons for screening as well as the risks and uncertainties. My colleagues and I have demonstrated that significant information about screening can be imparted in brief, easily understood disclosure statements.[35, 36] Greater understanding on the part of consumers will reduce the chances of malpractice suits, but, most important, it will increase the chances that testing will serve their best interests.

REFERENCES

1. Bickel, H. J., W. Gerrard, and E. M. Hickman. 1954. Influence of phenylalanine intake on the chemistry and behavior of a phenylketonuric child. Acta Paediat. 43:64–77.
2. Baumeister, A. A. 1967. The effects of dietary control on intelligence in phenylketonuria. Am. J. Ment. Defic. 71:840–847.
3. Holtzman, N. A., R. A. Kronmal, W. van Doorninck, C. Azen, and R. Koch. 1986. Effect of age at loss of dietary control on intellectual performance and behavior of children with phenylketonuria. N. Eng. J. Med. 314:593–598.
4. Tourian, A., and J. B. Sidbury. 1983. Phenylketonuria and hyperphenylalaninemia. Pp. 270–286 in The Metabolic Basis of Inherited Disease, J. B. Stanbury, J. B. Wyngaarden, D. S. Fredrickson, J. L. Goldstein, and M. S. Brown, eds. New York: McGraw-Hill.
5. Guthrie, R., and A. Susi. 1963. A simple phenylalanine method for detecting phenylketonuria in large populations of newborn infants. Pediatrics 32:338–343.
6. Holtzman, N. A. 1977. Anatomy of a trial. Pediatrics 60:932–934.
7. Holtzman, N. A., E. D. Mellits, and A. G. Meek. 1974. Neonatal screening for phenylketonuria. I. Effectiveness. JAMA 229:667–670.
8. Holtzman, N. A. 1970. Dietary treatment of inborn errors of metabolism. Ann. Rev. Med. 21:335–356.
9. Holtzman et al. 1974; see note 7.
10. Starfield, B., and N. A. Holtzman. 1975. A comparison of effectiveness of screening for phenylketonuria in the United States, United Kingdom and Ireland. N. Eng. J. Med. 293:118–121.
11. Holtzman et al. 1974; see note 7.
12. Ambrose, J. A. 1973. Report on a cooperative study of various fluorometric procedures and the Guthrie bacterial inhibition assay in the determination of hyperphenylalaninemia. Health Lab. Sci. 10:180–187.
13. Committee for the Study of Inborn Errors of Metabolism (CSIEM). 1975. Genetic Screening: Programs, Principles, and Research. Washington, D.C.: National Academy of Sciences.
14. Starfield and Holtzman. 1975; see note 10.
15. Holtzman, C., W. E. Slazyk, J. F. Cordero, and W. H. Hannon. 1986. Descriptive epidemiology of missed cases of phenylketonuria and congenital hypothyroidism. Pediatrics 1985. 78:553–558.
16. Andrews, L. B., ed. 1985. Legal Liability and Quality Assurance in Newborn Screening. Chicago: American Bar Foundation.
17. Brock, D. J. H., A. E. Bolton, and J. B. Scrimegeour. 1974. Prenatal diagnosis of spina bifida and anencephaly through maternal plasma-alpha-fetoprotein measurement. Lancet 1:767–769.
18. Holtzman, N. A. In press. Genetic variation in nutrition requirements and susceptibility to disease: Policy implications. Am. J. Clin. Nutr.
19. Report of Collaborative Acetylcholinesterase Study. 1981. Amniotic fluid acetylcholinesterase electrophoresis as a secondary test in the diagnosis of anencephaly and open spina bifida in early pregnancy. Lancet 2:321–326.

20. Office of Technology Assessment, U.S. Congress. 1988. Healthy Children: Investing in the Future. OTA-t-345. Washington, D.C.: Government Printing Office, pp. 93–116.
21. Meister, S. B., D. S. Shepard, and R. Zeckhauser. 1987. Cost effectiveness of prenatal screening for neural tube defects. Pp. 66–93 in Prenatal Screening, Policies, and Values: The Example of Neural Tube Defect, E. O. Nightingale and S. B. Meister, eds. Cambridge, Mass.: Harvard University Press.
22. Holtzman, N. A., R. R. Faden, C. O. Leonard, G. A. Chase, A. J. Chwalow, and S. Richmond. Submitted for publication. Effect of education on physicians' knowledge of a new technology: The case of alpha-fetoprotein screening for fetal neural tube defects.
23. Ibid.
24. Young, F. E. 1987. DNA probes; fruits of the new biotechnology. JAMA 258:2404–2406.
25. Holtzman, N. A. 1983. Prenatal screening for neural tube defects. Pediatrics 71:658–659.
26. Sun, M. 1983. FDA draws criticism on prenatal test. Science 221:440–442.
27. Annas, G. J., and S. Elias. 1985. Maternal serum AFP: Educating physicians and the public. Am. J. Public Health 75:1374–1375.
28. Lustig, L., S. Clarke, G. Cunningham, R. Schonberg, and G. Tomkinson. In press. California experience with low MSAFP results. Am. J. Med. Genet.
29. DiMaio, M. S., A. Baumgarten, R. M. Greenstein, H. M. Sasi, and M. J. Mahoney. 1987. Screening for fetal Down's syndrome in pregnancy by measuring maternal serum alpha-fetoprotein levels. N. Eng. J. Med. 317:342–346.
30. Holtzman et al. Submitted for publication.
31. Holtzman, N. A. In press. Proceed with Caution: Predicting Genetic Risks in the Recombinant DNA Era. Baltimore, Md.: Johns Hopkins University Press.
32. Office of Technology Assessment, U.S. Congress. 1988. The commercial development of tests for human genetic disorders. Health Program staff paper. Washington, D.C.
33. Ibid.
34. Andrews, L. B. 1987. Medical Genetics: A Legal Frontier. Chicago: American Bar Foundation.
35. Holtzman, N. A., R. Faden, A. J. Chwalow, and S. D. Horn. 1983. Effect of informed parental consent on mothers' knowledge of newborn screening. Pediatrics 72:807–812.
36. Faden, R. R., A. J. Chwalow, E. Orel-Crosby, N. A. Holtzman, G. A. Chase, and C. O. Leonard. 1985. What participants understand about a maternal serum alpha-fetoprotein screening program. Am. J. Public Health 75:1381–1384.

Effects on Access to and Delivery of Obstetrical Care

Obstetrical Care for Low-Income Women: The Effects of Medical Malpractice on Community Health Centers

DANA HUGHES, M.P.H., M.S., SARA ROSENBAUM, J.D., DAVID SMITH, M.D., AND CYNTHIA FADER, B.S.N.

The field of obstetrics has undergone intense and rapid change in recent years, in large part because of the crisis in professional liability. Rising premiums for malpractice insurance and escalating numbers of lawsuits have transformed obstetrics for providers and patients alike. Among the most dramatic changes has been the exodus of obstetricians and family doctors from obstetrical practice. Studies show that as many as 12 percent of obstetricians and 60 percent of family doctors have elected to omit obstetrics from their medical practices for malpractice-related reasons.[1, 2] Many more have decreased the number of deliveries they will perform for medically high-risk patients. The American College of Obstetricians and Gynecologists (ACOG) estimates that as many as 14 percent of obstetricians have decreased the number of their deliveries and 23 percent have decreased the percentage of their practice time devoted to high-risk obstetrics.[3]

These malpractice-driven reductions in obstetrical services are occurring at a time when the number of practicing obstetrical providers may already be poised to decrease, for three reasons. First, the "graying" of America is reducing the need for obstetrical services and increasing the need for gynecological care. The issue of professional liability is fueling this process.

Second, the number of uninsured and publicly insured women has increased substantially in recent years. Census data show that, between 1980 and 1985, the number of Americans under the age of 65 without health insurance grew by 40 percent.[4] By 1985, there were 14.5 million women of childbearing age without health insurance that covered maternity care and 9.5 million such women without any health insurance at all.[5]

In response to this problem Congress has greatly expanded the Medicaid program in recent years to cover more low-income women who otherwise would be uninsured, substantially increasing the number of publicly insured women. Nevertheless, the U.S. General Accounting Office (GAO) found in a recent study that women covered by Medicaid at the time of delivery are only slightly more likely than uninsured women to receive early care.[6] Several factors explain this phenomenon. The unwieldy Medicaid enrollment process alone can prevent a woman from receiving care until well into her pregnancy.[7] Another clear contributing factor is the relatively small percentage of obstetricians who will accept Medicaid patients. Only 63 percent of obstetricians reported that they take any Medicaid patients; of those who do, most see only a small number.[8] The average obstetrician who accepts Medicaid devotes about 8.3 percent of his or her patient load—approximately 12 patients a year[9]—to Medicaid beneficiaries.

The extent to which women are uninsured or publicly insured is especially important in a discussion of the delivery of maternity care because of the pivotal role that health insurance plays in the accessibility of care. The GAO found that less than one-third of uninsured women received adequate prenatal care, compared with 81 percent of insured women.[10] As a declining proportion of women of childbearing age are insured, obstetricians' ability and willingness to practice an expensive form of medicine are also likely to decline.

A third factor that contributes to the declining availability of obstetrical providers is the changing demographics of childbearing, which is increasingly concentrated among young, low-income, poorly educated women who, as a group, represent an unattractive patient load.[11] Obstetricians may be subconsciously, if not consciously, responding to this trend.

Although the availability of obstetrical providers has declined in recent years for all women, there has always been inadequate care for poor women. For example, much is made of obstetricians' "growing" unwillingness to accept Medicaid patients; in fact, the pool of obstetricians participating in the program shrank only slightly between 1977 and 1986, from 64 percent to about 63 percent. Indeed, a critical obstetrical shortage for poor women had been recognized by 1972 when the National Health Service Corps was created to deploy providers in underserved communities. At that time, priority was given to the placement of maternity care providers because of the critical shortage in many communities of obstetricians available and willing to serve low-income women. In short the exodus of physicians from obstetrical care generally, and from the care of low-income women specifically, exacerbates what was already a serious problem.

MEDICAL MALPRACTICE AND LOW-INCOME WOMEN

The threat of malpractice litigation and the high cost of liability insurance impose two strains—one direct and one indirect—on the obstetrical system. The direct strain is the cessation of practice among providers unwilling to expose themselves to suit. The indirect strain comes as the price of care is driven so high by escalating insurance premiums that it becomes unaffordable. Poor women are the most likely to be affected by the decline in availability because they cannot afford to pay the escalating rates. Moreover, as a result of their poverty, their insufficient food and poor nutrition, and lifetimes of inadequate health care, low-income women as a rule are at greater social and medical risk of pregnancy-related complications. Therefore, to the extent that obstetricians elect to limit their practice to low-risk patients, low-income women are, by definition, excluded.

Medicaid-covered patients and other low-income women are also unappealing as patients because providers cannot pass increased costs along to them. Medicaid reimbursement rates, which are always low in comparison with prevailing rates, are further eroded by rising malpractice insurance premiums—so much so that few doctors can afford to take many Medicaid patients.[12] In at least eight states malpractice insurance premiums per delivery are higher than global Medicaid fees paid to physicians for prenatal and delivery care.[13] Self-paying patients pose similar problems for doctors because most uninsured patients are unable to meet normal physician charges, let alone increases related to rising insurance premiums.

Physicians' fears of malpractice suits have disproportionately affected access to care for poor women because of a widely held but unsubstantiated perception among physicians that poor women are more litigious than nonpoor women.[14] Physicians who do not serve Medicaid patients report that this perceived litigiousness is among the principal reasons for their not taking Medicaid patients.[15]

Data are limited on the extent to which this crisis has affected care for low-income pregnant women, although the data that are available suggest that poor women may be less rather than more likely to pursue a malpractice incident.[16] There is ample documentation that providers who are able or willing to serve uninsured and publicly insured pregnant women are in limited supply, but these data do not always distinguish the influence of fear of malpractice suits from the influence of other factors, such as low reimbursement rates, slow payment, racial biases, and so on.[17]

PURPOSE OF STUDY

The purpose of this study was to determine the direct and indirect effects of the medical malpractice phenomenon—including rising premium rates, the escalating number of claims against obstetricians, and perceptions of increased risk of malpractice suits by poor women—on the availability of maternity services for low-income pregnant women at Community and Migrant Health Centers. Located in federally designated medically underserved areas, Community and Migrant Health Centers receive federal grants to furnish medical care to persons unable to obtain care from other sources. Health centers are explicitly designed to provide free and reduced-cost care to uninsured and low-income patients.

Health centers were selected as the subject of the study for three reasons. First, they are a major source of health care for low-income pregnant women. Of the 5.5 million people served by health centers in fiscal year 1986, approximately 1.3 million were women of childbearing age. That year, the centers provided maternity care to 120,000 pregnant women, more than half of whom had family incomes below 100 percent of the federal poverty level.

Second, in numerous communities the health center is the only provider willing to accept Medicaid and uninsured patients. Thus, the extent to which health centers are affected by the medical malpractice situation may indicate the effects of the situation on low-income women generally. In other communities the health center is the *only* health resource; if malpractice concerns affect these centers, care for virtually the entire community is affected.

Third, health centers can be expected to play an even greater role in the provision of maternity care in the future. As states expand their Medicaid programs to cover more women, the number of pregnancies covered by Medicaid will increase. In Washington State alone it is estimated that by 1995 one-third of all births will be to Medicaid-covered mothers, in contrast to 17 percent of all births in 1984–1985.[18] Without an increase in the pool of obstetricians who are willing to accept Medicaid patients, current providers, such as Community Health Centers, will have to accommodate this increased demand.

In analyzing the impact of the malpractice phenomenon we were mindful of the wide variations in staffing configurations in health centers. Staffing patterns range from full complements of staff professionals (obstetricians, family doctors, midwives, nurse-practitioners, and allied personnel) working at centers that are formally affiliated with hospitals, to contractual arrangements with private doctors, hospitals, and other providers of maternity care at center sites comparable to community general medical practices without staff specialists. The capacity of the staffs and the strength of the contractual arrangements determine the availability, accessibility, and quality of care that centers can provide.

We hypothesized that the malpractice climate—especially rising insurance premiums and the threat of litigation—may have reduced the centers' capacity to provide maternity care in various ways. First, centers that have their own obstetrical staff would be affected as the cost of maintaining that staff rose precipitously with escalating insurance premiums. Second, centers that contract for services would either lose contractors because of the contractors' malpractice concerns or else find themselves unable to afford the prices contractors charge to cover their increasing costs.

Health centers are expected to be especially vulnerable to the economic fallout of the malpractice problem: after deep cuts in their federal funding in 1981, they experienced modest increases until fiscal year 1988, when funding was frozen.[19] These increases did not offset the rising costs of providing care. Congress's Office of Technology Assessment found that the level of financial support in 1984 was less in real dollars than it had been four years earlier.[20] Furthermore, a steep rise in the proportion of uninsured persons occurred during the same time period. We surmised that these two trends—declining financial support and increased demand—would leave health centers unable to absorb rising costs and weather the malpractice storm.

Adding to the health centers' vulnerability is the virtual demise of the National Health Service Corps, which over the years has placed thousands of primary care physicians, including obstetricians, in areas in which there was a shortage of health manpower; most often, these physicians staffed health centers. Federal budget reductions, justified by a projected surplus of 50,000 physicians by 1990, resulted in a decline from 6,409 new corps scholarships in 1980 to 49 in 1987.[21]

METHODOLOGY

Data for this study were gathered in a survey of Community and Migrant Health Center directors during April and May 1988. A random sample of 208 centers was selected, representing 37 percent of all centers. Of the 208 questionnaires in the original sample, 69 were ultimately excluded because the respondents were not Community Health

Centers.[22] Thus, the actual sample size was 139, or 25 percent of all federally funded health centers.

Centers were mailed a six-page questionnaire and given the opportunity of answering either by telephone or by mail. Most responded by mail. Follow-up calls to clarify answers or to complete missing data were conducted for the majority of centers. Fifty-eight completed questionnaires were received, representing 42 percent of the sample.

Table 1 compares the distribution of health centers responding to the survey and the total distribution of centers by U.S. Public Health Service region; the percentages are similar. Likewise, responding centers reflected overall distributions of size and annual number of patients (Table 2).

Although the responses resemble the true distribution and size of all health centers, it is possible that the sample may be limited by a selection bias. Among the questions asked of the centers was whether a medical malpractice claim had ever been made against them. Some centers that have actually experienced such claims may have elected not to complete the survey. In that case our sample would represent a disproportionate number of centers without claims, whereas centers

TABLE 1 Distribution of Total and Responding Health Centers, by Region, 1988

Public Health Service Region	Total Centers		Responding Centers	
	Number	Percentage	Number	Percentage
I (Me., Vt., N.H., Mass., Conn., R.I.)	37	7	5	9
II (N.Y., N.J.)[a]	50	9	3	5
III (Pa., Va., W.Va., Md., Del., D.C.)	74	13	4	7
IV (Ky., Tenn., N.C., Miss., Ala., Ga., S.C., Fla.)	139	25	17	29
V (Minn., Wis., Mich., Ill., Ind., Ohio)	64	12	6	10
VI (N.M., Tex., Okla., Ark., La.)	53	10	9	16
VII (Neb., Iowa, Kans., Mo.)	23	4	2	3
VIII (Mont., N.D., S.D., Wyo., Utah, Colo.)	31	6	3	5
IX (Calif., Nev., Ariz., Hawaii)[b]	48	9	6	10
X (Wash., Ore., Idaho, Alaska)	27	5	1	2
Unknown	—	—	2	3
Total	546[c]	100	58	99

[a]Excludes Puerto Rico and the U.S. Virgin Islands.
[b]Excludes Guam and American Samoa.
[c]There are 568 centers in the United States and its territories. This figure excludes those located in Puerto Rico, the Virgin Islands, Guam, and American Samoa.
Total percentage does not equal 100 due to rounding.

TABLE 2   Distribution of Total and Responding
Health Centers, by Number of Encounters, 1987

Number of Encounters	Total Centers		Responding Centers	
	Number[a]	Percentage	Number	Percentage
< 4,999	226	41	19	33
5,000–9,000	170	31	14	24
10,000–14,999	77	14	11	19
> 15,000	69	13	12	21
Unknown	4[b]	1	2	3
Total	546	100	58	100

[a] There are 568 centers in the United States and its territories. This figure excludes those located in Puerto Rico, the Virgin Islands, Guam, and American Samoa.

[b] No female users aged 15–44 years.

with claims would be underrepresented. If so, the data from this survey on the severe difficulties of health centers become even more troubling because the responses would not include centers that have actually experienced malpractice litigation.

RESULTS

The vast majority of health centers reported that medical malpractice issues either directly or indirectly affected the provision of maternity care. Thirty-nine centers (67 percent) indicated that the medical malpractice phenomenon has affected either their ability to furnish obstetrical services or the scope of services they could offer. Nineteen of the centers (33 percent) reported that they were unaffected (Tables 3 and 4).

Of the 19 centers reporting no problems, most had some protection against financial and provider drain. Four were affiliated with hospitals and received medical malpractice insurance coverage through them. Two indicated that their doctors were commissioned officers of the U.S. Public Health Service and thus were either covered under the Federal Tort Claims Act or had their malpractice insurance paid for by the federal government. Four offered no maternity care at all, either because they were too small to justify establishing the service or because there were free services available in the community to which they could refer patients. Therefore, only 9 of the 19 centers (16 percent of total respondents) that reported themselves to be unaffected by the malpractice situation had no obvious protection against its high financial and professional costs. Of these 9 centers, most reported that they expected to be affected soon. "We are very fortunate," one center wrote, "but there is no question that [malpractice] represents a very serious problem."

TABLE 3 Malpractice Problems Among Responding Health Centers, by Region, 1987

Public Health Service Region	Total	Respondents (N = 58) Malpractice Posed Problems	Malpractice Did Not Pose Problems
I (Me., Vt., N.H., Mass., Conn., R.I.)	5	4	1
II (N.Y., N.J.)[a]	3	0	3
III (Pa., Va., W.Va., Md., Del., D.C.)	4	3	1
IV (Ky., Tenn., N.C., Miss., Ala., Ga., S.C., Fla.)	17	12	5
V (Minn., Wis., Mich., Ill., Ind., Ohio)	6	5	1
VI (N.M., Tex., Okla., Ark., La.)	9	4	5
VII (Neb., Iowa, Kans., Mo.)	2	1	1
VIII (Mont., N.D., S.D., Wyo., Utah, Colo.)	3	3	0
IX (Calif., Nev., Ariz., Hawaii)[b]	6	5	1
X (Wash., Ore., Idaho, Alaska)	1	0	1
Unknown	2	2	0
Total	58	39	19

[a] Excludes Puerto Rico and the U.S. Virgin Islands.
[b] Excludes Guam and American Samoa.

The professional liability climate affected health centers in two major ways: (1) by reducing their capacity to furnish or purchase maternity care through staff or contract providers and (2) by forcing some centers, as a result of certain practices in insurance policy writing, to furnish care that might ultimately place the centers at greater risk for malpractice suits. The net effect was to curtail access to maternity care for low-income women and in some areas to force centers to make practice decisions based on the requirements of insurance carriers rather than on standards of quality medical practice.

TABLE 4 Adverse Effects of Malpractice Costs Among Responding Health Centers, 1988

Effect	Respondents (N = 58) Number	Percentage
Limited number of physicians under contract	19	33
Hampered recruitment and retention of physicians	25	43
Limited number of physicians hired	26	45
Reduced number of maternity patients seen	26	45

Service Capacity

As noted earlier, most responding health centers provided some maternity care (either prenatal care alone or both prenatal and delivery services). Services were provided in several configurations: 21 centers (36 percent) reported that they offered maternity care through a combination of staff and contract providers; 12 (21 percent) said that they contracted out all maternity care; and 13 said they had sufficient staff to furnish all maternity care (Table 5).

Only 22 of the 34 centers with maternity care providers on staff indicated that the providers included obstetricians. Of these 22 centers, 15 (65 percent) reported that the doctors were assigned to them through the National Health Service Corps; only 7 had full- or part-time staff obstetricians that had *not* been acquired through the federal government. Thirteen centers used family physicians on staff for maternity care, either alone or in concert with contract physicians for backup or referral. Only 10 centers reported using midwives or midlevel practitioners for maternity care.

Affected centers reported that their existing maternity care systems were threatened or weakened because rising medical malpractice insurance costs or the specter of litigation, or both, limited their ability to recruit and retain staff or to establish and maintain contractual arrangements.

Provider Recruitment and Retention

Since their inception, Community and Migrant Health Centers have had difficulty recruiting and retaining physicians because of the relatively low salaries they must pay, their isolated locations, and the

TABLE 5 Arrangements for Providing Maternity Care Among Responding Health Centers, 1987

Arrangement	Respondents ($N = 58$)	
	Number	Percentage
Contract part of services	21	36
All salaried staff	13	22
Contract all services	12	21
No obstetrical care	6[a]	10
Referring for delivery without formal contract	5	9
Did not respond to question	1	2
Total	58	100

[a] Of these, three have informal referral arrangements for pregnant patients, and three do not.

intense work demanded of employees. The National Health Service Corps was established in large part because health centers and other providers in medically underserved areas had difficulty attracting staff. Although the corps provides a temporary remedy for health centers, it addresses only one aspect of the centers' recruitment problem at best: a potential pool of physicians. To recruit and retain corps assignees or any other staff, centers must also have the resources to pay competitive salaries. Over the years, most centers have managed to scrape together the funds needed to recruit corps assignees and other persons. However, the rising cost of malpractice insurance has cut deeply into the resources available for compensation, so much so that many centers are unable to provide all aspects of perinatal care and are unable to piece together a financial package that is adequate to retain recruited staff.

Twenty-five (46 percent) of the 54 responding centers that reported furnishing maternity care stated that the high cost of medical malpractice insurance limited their ability to recruit and retain maternity care providers. Moreover, the high cost of obstetrical care was a key factor in centers' decisions to offer no such care at all. Some centers stated that the rising premium rates being demanded for obstetrical providers were simply unaffordable. For other centers, malpractice insurance costs cut so deeply into their total compensation package that they could not offer competitive salaries and benefits.

Thirty-three of the responding centers reported no problems recruiting doctors; however, 38 percent of these centers were staffed exclusively with doctors from the National Health Service Corps. With the planned demise of the corps (the last 100 obligated scholars will be placed in 1994), the protection provided these centers by the corps will not last long.

Ironically, four centers indicated that malpractice problems made recruitment and retention of staff easier. These centers were all affiliated with hospitals; thus, their ability to offer malpractice insurance as a benefit through the hospital was a major incentive for physicians to work for them.

Contractual Arrangements

Community and Migrant Health Centers commonly contract with other providers for services that cannot be furnished on site. Twenty-one (36 percent) of the responding centers indicated that they contracted with local providers for some maternity services. Twelve centers (21 percent) contracted for all of their maternity services (see Table 5).

Contracting arrangements were established either to provide specialized backup or to supplement family practice physicians and midwives on staff. Of those centers that reported contracting for some or all of their maternity care, most did so because their family doctors or midwives were not allowed to attend deliveries. Because we did not ask specifically why family doctors could not attend deliveries, the reasons why centers contracted for maternity services are unclear; however, some centers volunteered that they could not afford the additional insurance costs required for coverage of delivery services. In some cases it appeared that hospitals refused to extend admitting privileges to family practitioners and midwives, thereby curtailing the ability of health center staff to deliver even low-risk patients.

Effect on Access to Maternity Care

The most profound effect of the malpractice phenomenon revealed through the survey was its impact on access to maternity care. Twenty-five centers (43 percent) indicated that they were forced to "turn patients away" because they were understaffed and were unable to recruit or contract with enough maternity care providers. The centers either could not afford the additional costs associated with treating these patients or could find no contract providers willing to affiliate with them. Most (17) of these centers were able to serve a portion of the patients who sought care but were forced to deny care to others.

Centers indicated that patients who could not be served were generally given suggestions about where else they might obtain care, although some centers were unable to establish even informal referral arrangements with other providers. Several centers reported that they had no one to whom they could refer the patients they could not serve, either because private providers would not take the patients or because there were no alternative providers at all. One center indicated that there were no community doctors in the area who would accept Medicaid reimbursement. Another reported that patients with insurance were sent to the nearest obstetrician, 45 miles away; those without insurance were sent to the university hospital, 65 miles away.

Six responding centers were unable to provide care to any pregnant patient because they could neither provide care on site nor contract with other providers.* Of these six centers, five cited the high cost of providing obstetrical care, including rising medical malpractice insurance premiums, as the major reason for not offering maternity care. One

---

* Three of these centers used informal referral networks to suggest where pregnant patients might go but had no formal contractual system; the remaining three indicated that no such networks existed.

center put it bluntly, "We are unable to provide on-site or contract off-site prenatal care and delivery services because of the high cost of medical malpractice insurance. As a result, the center is offering none of these services."

Five centers (10 percent of the 52 centers furnishing maternity care) reported that they were forced to discontinue care of women at the time of delivery because the family doctors or midwives on staff could not perform deliveries and could not identify community physicians to whom they could refer patients for delivery care, either on a formal or informal basis. The patients were virtually on their own to locate delivery care. One center reported that it was forced to send all patients—nearly 700 a year—to the local hospital emergency room for deliveries. Another referred patients to the county hospital for deliveries.

Center providers were prohibited from delivering babies either because their malpractice insurance policies prohibited it or because local hospitals allowed deliveries only by obstetricians. In turn, the fear of malpractice suits and the rising costs of malpractice insurance were cited as the primary reasons for community obstetricians' unwillingness to contract with the centers or to accept referrals. One center wrote, "Only one in three obstetricians in the community does obstetrics [at all] because of the high cost of malpractice. And no family doctors do obstetrics because of lack of obstetrical backup."

Malpractice and Standards of Care

Ironically, the malpractice insurance system itself has created the risk of claims against some health centers through two avenues. First, family doctors and nurse-midwives were forced into the medically unsound practice of discontinuing care for patients at the time of delivery because they were unable to obtain community backup or referrals for delivery. This discontinuance of care could be characterized as abandonment, which constitutes grounds for liability and loss of license.

Second, some centers reported that they were forced to replace experienced doctors with new graduates because of the escalating malpractice premium costs for experienced physicians. Insurers base this practice on the theory of "accumulated exposure," that is, that the risk of being sued increases over time. Thus, patients were deprived of the most experienced physicians as a means of avoiding higher malpractice insurance costs.

Increased Risk for Family Doctors

As a matter of economy, most health centers with maternity care providers on staff employ family doctors rather than obstetricians. One-third of the centers reported that they were staffed with family practitioners who furnished prenatal care. However, as indicated above, the centers also reported that the vast majority of these physicians were not permitted to deliver babies because of insurance or hospital credentialing limitations. Family practice staff delivered babies in only 6 percent of the centers.

When family doctors and other providers have strong referral networks for delivery, this arrangement is not necessarily troublesome. Many centers in our survey, however, were unable to develop backup or referral arrangements, and the family doctors and midwives were placed in the untenable position of having to choose whether to drop the patient at the time of delivery (and hope that she could make it to the emergency room), deliver a baby without malpractice coverage, or cease furnishing prenatal care altogether. Ceasing care of the patient at the time of delivery not only places the patient in jeopardy and the physician in an ethical and liability dilemma but also creates potential liability for the physician who ultimately performs the delivery without any prior knowledge of the patient.

Accumulated Exposure

Data from the centers regarding the costs of malpractice insurance show that, among most of those reporting this information, rates have increased substantially in recent years (Table 6). The cost of coverage for obstetricians increased by more than 400 percent between 1985 and 1987 at one center and for family doctors by almost 150 percent at another. These increases apparently had little or nothing to do with claims experiences because only eight of the responding centers had ever had a maternity-related claim made against them.

One factor that did enter into the price determination, at least in some states, was provider experience. Seven centers reported that premium rates for young, newly credentialed doctors were lower than those for experienced physicians. Centers were told that this was because more experienced doctors, by virtue of their greater number of years in practice, were more likely to be sued. One center reported that the cost of malpractice insurance was almost three times higher for the doctor who had worked there for more than seven years than it was for a newly recruited doctor with less than two years of experience at the center. Another center, which was ultimately unsuccessful in recruiting an obstetrician, was told by its insurance company that the premium for a first-year obstetrician would be $30,000; over the next four years that premium would increase to $60,000. At this center, as at others, costs apparently leveled off after a physician had been employed there from five to eight years.

TABLE **6** Malpractice Insurance Costs per Practitioner at Responding Health Centers, 1985–1987[a]

1985 Costs ($)	1987 Costs ($)	Percent Increase
Obstetricians		
7,000	35,265	403
4,570	16,750	266
7,007	24,607	251
28,450	72,097	153
6,000	15,000	150
20,000	45,000	125
18,124	39,984	121
25,000	48,000	92
22,886	35,780	56
23,521	36,046	53
24,000	32,000	33
Family Practitioners		
3,251	8,042	147
1,700	4,200	147
4,200	8,600	105[b]
5,500	11,000	100
2,000	3,731	87
574	1,066	86
3,900	7,100	82[b]
7,194	12,132	69
4,869	6,908	42
6,700	8,400	25
8,000	9,000	13[b]
2,500	2,800	12[b]
Midwives		
585	4,088	599
1,498	1,605	7

[a] Includes all centers reporting these data.
[b] These practitioners provided prenatal care only. None was allowed to deliver babies under the insurance policy.

Per Se Risk

Some centers were unable to obtain insurance for any doctors delivering babies, even at an elevated price. One center was turned down by a company because, according to the insurance carrier, "center patients posed an inherent risk." In such cases, centers are placed in an impossible bind: they are unable to obtain insurance for either seasoned, experienced doctors or for young, inexperienced doctors.

CONCLUSIONS

Our survey of health centers confirms that, in addition to consequences documented elsewhere, the rapid escalation of medical malpractice premiums has taken a terrible toll on the number of medical care providers who are willing or able to serve low-income pregnant women. The vast majority of centers surveyed felt the impact of malpractice costs on the health services they offered. Nearly every center furnishing maternity care experienced a reduction in its ability to provide or purchase necessary health services for pregnant women. Many centers with adequate staff to furnish at least low-risk maternity care have been forced to curtail or eliminate services because insurers refuse to provide delivery coverage except at exorbitant costs that clinics cannot afford. Still other health centers have seen the disintegration of their referral arrangements to specialists as more and more obstetricians either leave the practice of obstetrics altogether or else refuse to treat those they perceive to be high-risk patients.

Several observations are in order. First, it is evident that, given the need for services and the scarcity of financial resources, the federal government cannot afford to have vast sums of public health money diverted into malpractice insurance. The U.S. Department of Health and Human Services estimates that in fiscal year 1988 approximately $30 million of the $445 million appropriation for health centers will be spent on malpractice insurance for health center staff. Much of this cost will be attributable to obstetrics-related activities. This $30 million expenditure on malpractice insurance represents 7 percent of the centers' total budget—sufficient funding to build about 60 health centers in medically underserved areas or to increase by one-third the funds now being spent by health centers on maternity care.

Second, this expenditure is particularly disturbing given the fact that there appears to be no relationship between the rapid escalation of costs and the centers' malpractice claims profiles. Only eight (14 percent) of the centers in our study had ever had a claim filed against them—far fewer than the average 73 percent of obstetrician-gynecologists in private practice who have been sued.[23] Although centers with more claims might not have responded to our survey, other studies confirm that physicians practicing in health centers have modest (16 percent) claims profiles.[24] Thus, for health centers, the adverse effects generated by malpractice premiums are particularly unwarranted.

Third, some insurers appear to be engaging in practices that we consider to be unconscionable. Physicians and midwives who are capable of attending at least low-risk pregnant women have been effectively disinsured for delivery services unless they pay astronomical rates. As referral providers simultaneously disappear, health centers are being forced to make inadequate, uncontrolled delivery arrangements for their patients—in some instances simply referring them to hospitals for delivery by house staff—rather than following patients through delivery themselves or through a carefully arranged network.

Other practices seriously compromise high-quality care. For example, the practice of penalizing experienced physicians constitutes a "your-number-is-up" approach to malpractice coverage. This policy means simply that health centers will be able to afford only relatively young, inexperienced physicians.

It is evident that such insurer practices do not promote comprehensive, high-quality care. Rates do not depend on adherence to carefully designed standards of quality, nor are they tied to experience, credentials, or continuing education. Instead, they constitute, in our opinion, a blatant attempt to shield companies from risk by discouraging or prohibiting physicians from engaging in the practice of obstetrics altogether. In short, malpractice insurers, by denying coverage to qualified center physicians, by discriminating against more experienced physicians, and by contributing to an overall reduction in the financial resources clinics have at their disposal, have succeeded in reducing the quality and availability of care received by center patients.

RECOMMENDATIONS

Based on our findings, we recommend two immediate, short-term reforms. First, all health center staff and contract providers engaged in obstetrical work should be brought under the protection of the Federal Tort Claims Act (FTCA). This move would save millions of dollars and provide immediate no-cost malpractice coverage. The FTCA currently insures both commissioned officers of the National Health Service Corps and National Health Service Corps scholarship graduates who work as civilian employees of the Public Health Service. Since 1984, health centers that employ corps physicians have paid some or all of their salaries with funds transferred to the centers by the service from the corps account. This fund transfer arrangement has cost corps members FTCA coverage simply because the name of the payer has been changed. Because the health center payer is a federal grantee and because the corps member compensated by the center is performing tasks identical to those performed by health service counterparts, there is no reason to discriminate between civilian and commissioned corps members employed by the health service and those employed by federal grantees. Moreover, there is no reason to distinguish among medical staff hired by federal grantees—indeed, legislation enacted as part of the fiscal year

1988 appropriations act eliminated the distinction between civilian contract physicians and physicians employed by the Indian Health Service and extended FTCA coverage to the former.[25]

By extending FTCA coverage to all medical and health staff working at health centers, the federal government would save tens of millions of dollars that could be reinvested in patient care. In an era of scarce financial resources, the government simply cannot afford to waste these funds. We recommend that the act cover not only National Health Service Corps assignees but also other medical and health staff employed by centers on a part- or full-time basis.

Second, we believe that a substantial expansion of the National Health Service Corps is warranted. Even if the immediate financial burden of malpractice insurance were lifted, clinics would continue to experience enormous difficulties in recruiting and retaining qualified personnel, given the areas and populations they serve. Moreover, although the most recent malpractice crisis has decreased the number of physicians willing to treat publicly insured or uninsured patients (the vast majority of health centers' patient populations), in fact the problem of nonparticipation in Medicaid and other public health programs by obstetricians may be only slightly greater than it was roughly a decade ago. Thus, the current crisis may be the result of continued high rates of nonparticipation accompanied by a shrinking pool of obstetricians. In sum, there continues to be a major need for corps personnel, particularly in the field of obstetrics. We recommend adding at least 500 physicians and another 250–500 midwives and other midlevel professionals. The savings generated by improved access to maternity care would more than pay for the outlay for personnel.

We believe that two long-term reforms are also required if the crisis in access to maternity care is to be remedied. First, we recommend the establishment of a national task force to draw up the elements of a no-fault system for obstetrics. The system would include not only a means for compensating patients but a means for overseeing and enforcing the quality of obstetrical care practiced in the United States. Whatever compensation poor women derive from the current malpractice system (and evidence suggests that they draw little in proportion to the incidents of substandard practice they suffer), both they and their children would benefit infinitely more from a well-regulated obstetrical system in which patient compensation was paid in the event of an unintended injury.

Second, we feel that no change of this magnitude can occur without significant reforms in the way physicians are licensed, credentialed, and monitored, and without uniform rules regarding the content of care and appropriate practice standards. As Law and Polan have observed in *Pain and Profit,* the medical care education system is national in scope, as are the standards of practice to which the public expects physicians to adhere.[26] Medical care no longer stops at state borders but is a vital national industry. It is essential, therefore, to call a halt to state-by-state regulation of the accreditation, content, and scope of obstetrical practice. By permitting individual states (and even individual hospitals) to establish their own qualifying and regulatory standards for physicians and midlevel professionals, the federal government has permitted an astonishing array of standards and practices to govern the scope and quality of obstetrical care.

The "locality rule," which held physicians to community rather than national standards of reasonable practice, died long ago in the nation's courtrooms, as Law and Polan have pointed out. It is essential that we lay to rest as well the locality system for regulating the practice of obstetrics. We believe the medical profession's failure to recognize the significance of the demise of the locality rule and its persistence in treating the regulation of medical practice as a local activity has caused part of the public mistrust that results in malpractice litigation. Thus, we recommend the development of national standards for obstetrical practice and for accreditation of physicians and midlevel professionals, as well as uniform monitoring and enforcement mechanisms. Otherwise, the stage simply cannot be set for the removal of obstetrics from the current malpractice system.

REFERENCES AND NOTES

1. American College of Obstetricians and Gynecologists (ACOG). 1985. Professional Liability Insurance and Its Effect: Report of a Survey of ACOG's Membership. Washington, D.C.
2. Health Care in Rural America: The Crisis Unfolds. 1988. Report to the Joint Task Force of the National Association of Community Health Centers and the National Rural Health Association. Washington, D.C., pp. 1–12.
3. ACOG. 1985; see note 1.
4. Sulvetta, M., and K. Swartz. 1986. The Uninsured and Uncompensated Care. Washington, D.C.: Urban Institute.
5. Gold, R., and A. Kenney. 1985. Paying for maternity care. Fam. Plan. Perspect. 17(May/June):103–111.
6. General Accounting Office (GAO), U.S. Congress. 1987. Prenatal Care: Medicaid Recipients and Uninsured Women Obtain Insufficient Care. GAO/HRD-87-137. Gaithersburg, Md.
7. Hill, I. 1988. Reaching Women Who Need Prenatal Care. Washington, D.C.: Center for Policy Research, National Governors' Association, p. 5.
8. American College of Obstetricians and Gynecologists (ACOG), Committee on Health Care for Underserved Women. 1988. OB/GYN Services for Indigent Women: Issues Raised by an ACOG Survey. Washington, D.C.

9. Mitchell, J., and J. Cromwell. 1983. Access to private physicians for public patients: Participation in Medicaid and Medicare. Pp. 105–129 in Securing Access to Health Care: The Ethical Implications of Differences in the Availability of Health Services. Washington, D.C.: President's Commission for the Study of Ethical Problems in Medicine and Biomedical and Behavioral Research.

10. GAO. 1987. Prenatal Care; see note 6.

11. Bureau of the Census, U.S. Department of Commerce. Issued annually. Fertility of American Women. Washington, D.C.: Government Printing Office.

12. Hughes, D., and S. Rosenbaum. 1987. Personal communication.

13. Ibid.

14. ACOG. 1988; see note 8.

15. Ibid.

16. General Accounting Office (GAO), U.S. Congress. 1987. Medical Malpractice: Characteristics of Claims Closed in 1984. GAO/HRD- 87-55. Gaithersburg, Md.

17. See, for example, Lazarus, W., and J. Tirengel. 1988. Back to Basics, 1988. Los Angeles: Southern California Child Health Network; Hoogesteger, J. 1987. Obstetricians extend time for indigents. Springfield News-Leader. June 23; Obstetricians' strike threat uses patients as pawns (editorial). 1987. Providence Journal. Feb. 10; County's delivery of babies almost extinct say doctors. 1987. Sequoyah County [Oklahoma]. April 12.

18. Peterson, J., Director of Policy, Washington State Medicaid Agency. 1988. Personal communication.

19. Children's Defense Fund. 1988. A Children's Defense Budget. Washington, D.C.

20. Office of Technology Assessment, U.S. Congress. 1988. Healthy Children: Investing in the Future. OTA-t-345. Washington, D.C.: Government Printing Office.

21. Gapen, P. 1988. The Health Service Corps: Endangered species? Med. Health Perspect. July 4.

22. The sample was selected from the membership list of the National Association of Community Health Centers, which includes all federally funded health centers plus a small proportion of nonproviders, such as individual members and state associations. Some nonproviders were selected in the initial random sample but were eliminated from the evaluation.

23. ACOG. 1985; see note 1.

24. National Association of Community Health Centers. 1986. The Medical Malpractice Claims Experience of Community and Migrant Health Centers. Washington, D.C.

25. Pub. L. 100-102, § 103(c).

26. Law, S., and S. Polan. 1978. Pain and Profit: The Politics of Malpractice. New York: Harper and Row.

Medical Professional Liability and Access to Obstetrical Care: Is There a Crisis?

DEBORAH LEWIS-IDEMA, M.SC.

The costs of professional liability insurance have risen dramatically in recent years. Between 1984 and 1987, premiums paid by the average obstetrician-gynecologist rose more than 70 percent—to $37,000 per year.[1] Family practitioners who provide obstetrical services pay almost twice as much for insurance as their colleagues who do not practice obstetrics.[2] Surveys by national and state organizations indicate that physicians are dropping the practice of obstetrics or changing the levels and types of care they render in response to malpractice concerns. Incidents of women who experience extreme difficulty in obtaining adequate maternity services have been reported throughout the United States.

The growing sense that there may be a crisis in obstetrical care has particular implications for low-income patients. There has been little improvement in infant and neonatal mortality rates in the United States in recent years, and the number of women receiving late or no prenatal care is large. Low-income patients, who face more barriers to access to care than more affluent patients, are also more likely to be medically at risk, to experience higher rates of infant mortality, and to have low-birthweight babies than more affluent patients. Residents of rural areas are also likely to encounter difficulty in obtaining care: a single physician's decision to stop practicing obstetrics can result in impaired access for women who have trouble reaching distant providers.

In this chapter I examine the relationship of professional liability issues and access to obstetrical care for low-income women and women living in rural areas. Drawing primarily on the numerous studies done by state and national organizations in the past several years, I attempt to determine whether the sense of crisis is justified and, if so, how the crisis might be addressed.

METHODOLOGY

Examining the relationship between professional liability concerns and access to care is like assembling a jigsaw puzzle. The research on this question is extremely limited, and there is no scientific study showing that the number of physicians serving low-income women is declining and that the decline is due to malpractice concerns. Various pieces of information from numerous sources must be drawn together to obtain a picture, or at least an outline, of the situation.

For this report, I reviewed 30 state studies, principally from state and national medical associations,[3] and nine national studies.[4] The available literature highlights the impact of professional liability concerns on physician decisions to provide obstetrical care; only a few studies examine access to care directly. The studies vary enormously in extensiveness and methodology. Some are highly rigorous, whereas others are simple, one-page questionnaires; most are descriptive. Response rates also vary significantly.

The most important caution regarding the research is that in a number of cases questions were asked in a manner that presupposed the answer. Almost all of the studies sought to determine whether physicians were changing their practices as a result of professional liability concerns. Many studies, however, phrased the question as "Have you changed your practice due to malpractice concerns (or the malpractice crisis)?" This phraseology does not distinguish between situations in which physicians ceased practicing obstetrics because of age, health, or simply boredom and those in which professional liability concerns were their predominant motivation. It is likely that any physician who discontinued, curtailed, or altered obstetrical practice in the last four or five years can reasonably attribute the decision to malpractice concerns, but there may have been other motivating factors as well. Studies that ask the question in two parts—"Have you changed practice? If so, why?"—are more likely to separate malpractice from nonmalpractice motivations.

Although the available literature may tend to overstate the importance of malpractice considerations in physicians' decision making, such overstatement does not mean the literature should be discarded. As a whole the studies document trends that appear to be influenced by physicians' malpractice concerns. Equally important, the absence of conclusive proof does not obviate the need for policy consideration of the issues surrounding malpractice and access. If there is good reason to believe that access to obstetrical care for low-income women and rural women is being affected by malpractice concerns, to wait for accurate, statistically valid studies would be highly inappropriate.

PROFESSIONAL LIABILITY CONCERNS AND CHANGING OBSTETRICAL PRACTICE

Several logically related questions must be examined to determine whether professional liability concerns are affecting access to care. To provide a framework for analyzing the widely varying state studies, I arrayed the states on each of the reported variables and constructed a median state.

What Changes Are Occurring in Obstetrical Practice?

The literature indicates that sizable numbers of obstetrical providers—both obstetrician-gynecologists (ob-gyns) and family practitioners—are eliminating obstetrics from their practice, reducing care to identifiable high-risk populations, or reducing the overall number of deliveries they perform (Table 1).

• Elimination of obstetrics: The American College of Obstetricians and Gynecologists (ACOG) reports that in 1987 12.4 percent of its members stopped practicing obstetrics as a result of professional liability concerns; the state surveys report that from 7 to 70 percent of responding physicians have stopped. In the median state, 25 percent of all surveyed obstetrical providers have stopped practicing obstetrics. The studies that surveyed ob-gyns alone report that from 6 to 30 percent of respondents stopped obstetrical practice. In the median state, 17 percent of ob-gyns reported eliminating obstetrics.

The attrition rate among family practitioners is higher than that among ob-gyns. The American Academy of Family Physicians (AAFP) reported that, by the end of 1985, 23.3 percent of its members—twice the proportion reported by the ACOG—had stopped practicing obstetrics because of malpractice concerns. The state studies reported that from 8 to 75 percent of family practitioners had dropped obstetrics over the past five years. Seven of the studies allowed direct comparison of changes between family practitioners and ob-gyns. In only one (Maryland) was the proportion of family practitioners stopping obstetrics smaller than the proportion of ob-gyns stopping this part of their practice.

TABLE 1   Summary Data (as percentage) from Studies of
Professional Liability and Obstetrical Practice

Range	Eliminated Obstetrics		Reduced High-Risk Care	Reduced Volume
	All Phys.	OB-GYNs		
All Studies				
	$N = 33$	$N = 17$	$N = 11$	$N = 13$
Minimum	7.00	5.90	16.00	5.80
Maximum	75.00	30.00	48.70	28.00
Median	25.00	14.30	23.60	12.90
State Studies				
	$N = 27$	$N = 14$	$N = 8$	$N = 8$
Minimum	7.00	5.90	16.00	5.80
Maximum	75.00	30.00	48.70	28.00
Median	25.00	17.50	24.30	18.50

• Reduced care for high-risk women: The state studies report that from 16 to 49 percent of ob-gyns reduced service to high-risk women. In the median state, almost one-quarter of ob-gyns reduced or eliminated service to this population. This figure is similar to that reported by the ACOG: in 1987, 27 percent of its members reduced or eliminated services to high-risk women.

• Reduced volume of obstetrical care: This is perhaps the most difficult practice change to document from the state studies. Only eight of them report on this subject, with 6 to 28 percent of physicians saying they were reducing the number of deliveries they perform. The median was 18.5 percent. By comparison, the ACOG reported that about 13 percent of member ob-gyns reduced their volume of care in 1987; the AAFP reports reductions by less than 10 percent of member family practitioners.

The state studies tend to show higher proportions of physicians altering their practice of obstetrics than do the ACOG and AAFP data. This disparity may reflect methodological differences among the state and national studies, but it may also reflect real geographic variation in physician behavior. It is logical to expect that studies would have been conducted in those states in which malpractice issues have been particularly critical to the profession.

Are These Changes Occurring Because of Professional Liability Concerns?

Physicians consistently report that they are reducing or eliminating their obstetrical practice because of the cost of malpractice insurance or

TABLE 2   Physicians Reporting Malpractice Issues as a Factor in Their Decision to Change Practice (as percentage)

Range	Studies ($N = 16$) of All Physicians	Studies ($N = 13$) of Physicians Who Changed Practice
Minimum	9.10	18.60
Maximum	70.00	99.00
Median	24.15	57.00

the risk of being sued. Although the precise numbers reported should be viewed with caution, the direction of these responses is too compelling to discount as an artifact of survey construction.

• Twenty-nine studies report that between 9 and 99 percent of all physicians surveyed have changed their obstetrical practice because of professional liability issues. The studies were subdivided into those reporting on all physicians and those reporting on physicians who had made practice changes. In the median state, more than half of the physicians who changed their practice said that malpractice concerns were a major factor in their decision (Table 2).

• In studies in which the question of motivation was separated from the act of changing obstetrical practices, *professional liability issues were cited by more than half the respondents as a major determinant in their decision to change.* In Georgia, for instance, 55 percent of ob-gyns dropping obstetrics cited malpractice concerns as the sole reason for their decision. In Illinois, 57 percent cited malpractice insurance costs and 44 percent cited the risk of being sued. In Kentucky, 78 percent of family physicians stopping obstetrics and 38 percent of those reducing their caseloads cited malpractice concerns.

• Studies of family practitioners have tended to provide respondents with the broadest range of choices for describing their motivation. These studies show a greater influence of personal factors—but malpractice concerns are of equal or greater importance. Although the Alabama, Ohio, and Washington reports found that 25 to 50 percent of respondents cited personal or professional concerns (age, health, time, lack of alternative physician coverage), 50 to 70 percent of respondents cited malpractice issues as a key factor in their decision.

• Only one study (Ohio) included statistical tests on the relationship between malpractice concerns and the decision to stop practicing obstetrics. The relationship was found to be statistically significant.

Summary

It is clear that major changes are occurring in the practice of obstetrics. A sizable number of physicians are eliminating or reducing obstetrical services and reducing services to high-risk women. Most physicians cite malpractice-related issues as a principal factor in their decision.

Certainly, the importance of malpractice concerns as the sole determinant of physician behavior may be overstated. Even apart from the wording of questionnaires, the current climate, both within the profession and among the public, is one in which the "malpractice crisis" is accepted as a rational explanation for the decision to stop or reduce provision of obstetrical services. For some physicians who are considering changing their practice for personal reasons, malpractice may simply be the factor that finally tips the balance. Nevertheless, the sheer weight of reports from physicians indicates the importance of malpractice concerns in their decisions to eliminate or reduce obstetrical care.

THE IMPACT OF PHYSICIAN PRACTICE CHANGES ON ACCESS TO CARE

Only nine of the state studies specifically sought information on the impact of changes in physician practice on access to care. Relevant information is also available from state agencies and national studies and from research that has looked specifically at changes in rural areas.

Access for Medicaid Recipients and Low-Income Women

All of the studies that asked physicians specifically about care for low-income patients reported declines in provider participation.

- In Illinois, 17 percent of physicians practicing obstetrics plan to reduce participation in Medicaid. Almost two-thirds of Washington ob-gyns limit the number of Medicaid patients they serve. In West Virginia, 41 percent of ob-gyns (compared with an average of 18 percent for all physicians) report that they do not serve Medicaid patients owing to liability concerns.
- Almost 13 percent of Oregon obstetrical practitioners stopped serving Medicaid patients during 1986–1987; another one-third specifically limit their Medicaid caseloads. About 10 percent have recently stopped providing charity care, and more than 40 percent limit the charity care they provide.
- Only 45 percent of Kentucky physicians serve Medicaid obstetrical patients. Three-quarters of the physicians who have reduced their provision of obstetrical care cite malpractice issues as a reason for nonparticipation in Medicaid. Only one-third of Maryland ob-gyns accept Medicaid.

• In January 1987, 133 physicians in Denver provided obstetrical services to Medicaid patients; the state Medicaid program reported that, by December of that year, only 9 (apart from hospital-based personnel) were still providing such care. In the entire state of Colorado, only 46 primary care physicians were accepting Medicaid obstetrical patients in December 1987.[5]

• In Texas, indigent women on average constitute 10 percent of the ob-gyn caseload. About one-third of ob-gyns report that they are limiting indigent care "a great deal"; another one-third are not limiting care at all.

• More than half the ob-gyns in North Carolina had been providing services in local health departments. Almost 30 percent reported stopping because of malpractice concerns.

One effect of reduced physician involvement in Medicaid is that caseloads for those who continue to provide care are increasing. In Washington State, the average number of deliveries per Medicaid provider rose from 14.8 in fiscal year 1985 to 16.8 in fiscal year 1986. Although the number of participating ob-gyns actually increased slightly, the number of participating family and general practitioners fell by 9.3 percent. At the same time, the number of Medicaid deliveries increased. As a result, the average number of Medicaid deliveries for ob-gyns rose from 26.4 in fiscal year 1985 to 28.3 in fiscal year 1986. For family physicians, the increase was from 7.5 to 8.3 deliveries (Table 3).

A recent National Governors' Association survey of state Medicaid and Maternal and Child Health agencies includes at least one response from each state (the District of Columbia did not respond). This report therefore may provide the broadest overview of the impact of malpractice concerns on access to care. According to the administrators of public programs, malpractice issues are reducing significantly the number of participating providers, and some areas of their states are experiencing major problems in access to care.[6]

• More than 60 percent of Medicaid programs and almost 90 percent of Maternal and Child Health programs are experiencing significant difficulty in finding providers who are willing to render maternity care. Nine out of ten programs say that rising malpractice insurance costs have contributed to this problem.

• Three-fifths of the agencies reported that physicians have stopped providing care to their clients because of malpractice concerns. Seven out of ten agencies said that the number of providers was decreasing for that reason.

TABLE 3 Changes in Deliveries by Medicaid Maternity Care
Providers in Washington State, 1985–1986

Deliveries	1985	1986	Change (%)
All providers[a]	858	821	−4.3
Mean number per provider	14.8	16.8	13.6
Percentage of providers with			
1–5 deliveries	53.3	50.2	−5.8
21+ deliveries	18.6	20.5	10.2
Obstetrician-gynecologists	235	246	4.7
Mean number per provider	26.4	28.3	7.3
Percentage of providers with			
1–5 deliveries	32.3	30.9	−4.3
21+ deliveries	35.3	37.4	5.9
Family general practitioners	345	313	−9.3
Mean number per provider	7.5	8.3	10.8
Percentage of providers with			
1–5 deliveries	53.6	59.1	10.2
21+ deliveries	7.5	8.0	6.0

[a] Includes clinics, midwives, and unidentified providers.
SOURCE: Washington Department of Social and Health Services. 1987. Maternity Care Access. Olympia.

- In response to an open-ended question, 21 states reported at least 484 counties in which low-income women, Medicaid recipients, or both have limited access to prenatal and delivery services. Because this information was not specifically requested in the questionnaire, responses may understate the extent of the problem.
- About half of the agencies regarded low reimbursement rates as the primary deterrent to provider participation in their programs. One-fifth considered malpractice insurance costs the most important reason.

Access to Care in Rural Areas

Family practitioners have traditionally been key providers of obstetrical care in rural areas. The high rates at which these physicians are leaving obstetrical practice appear to be generating significant access problems in some parts of the country.

- It is estimated, based on data from the AAFP and the ACOG, that the number of obstetrical providers in nonmetropolitan areas has fallen by about 20 percent over the past five years. This decline is particularly significant among family physicians (Figure 1).
- In 1986, 17 counties in Georgia had no obstetrical providers; there were only 25 physicians providing obstetrical care in all of rural Nevada.

One-third of Arizona's family physicians outside Maricopa and Pima counties (Phoenix and Tucson) had stopped providing obstetrical care by the end of 1985. In Idaho, more than one-quarter of ob-gyns have dropped obstetrics; in West Virginia, another largely rural state, more than half the ob-gyns have considered leaving the state.

• Rural physicians perceive a greater potential impact on access to care than do urban physicians. In California and Oregon, a greater proportion of rural physicians reported women without access to care. Although more physicians have stopped obstetrical practice in Detroit than in rural Michigan, 69 percent of rural physicians report access problems, compared with 61 percent in Detroit.

• A 1985 survey of small and rural California hospitals reported that 30 of 56 respondents providing obstetrical care had family physicians on their staff who were planning to drop obstetrics. Thirty-six of the hospitals (64 percent) indicated that they would cut back or eliminate their obstetrical services.

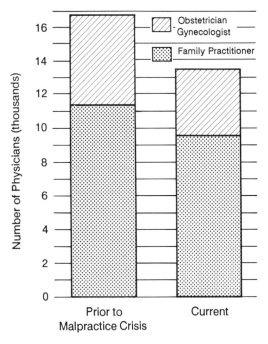

FIGURE 1 Changes in number of rural physicians practicing obstetrics.

• Sixty of the agencies responding to the National Governors' Association survey reported geographic areas with significant access problems—and 87 percent of these reported that the access problem was particularly acute in rural areas. Thirty-five of the 50 states reported problems with provider participation and access to care in rural areas.

Summary

As a whole, the literature suggests that professional liability concerns among physicians are generating access problems. In instances in which attrition from obstetrical practice has been great, caseloads for the remaining physicians increase, as suggested by the experience in Washington State. This trend creates a vicious circle, wherein physicians who continue to accept Medicaid patients experience greater pressures on their time—possibly to the point where they need to begin restricting their Medicaid practice. With fewer physicians providing obstetrical care, the low-income patient or Medicaid recipient, who may be perceived as less financially, socially, or medically desirable, can end up competing with a middle-class patient for the physician's time.

Although reduced availability of care for high-risk patients affects the entire population, it has particular implications for low-income women. These women are statistically more likely to be medically at risk and have higher rates of infant mortality and low-birthweight babies. This population requires easier access than the general population to the kind of care appropriate for high-risk mothers; yet that care appears to be less widely available to them.

Every study that looked at the relationship between malpractice concerns and Medicaid found that physicians report that they are reducing their Medicaid caseloads, at least in part, because of malpractice concerns. The state agencies, which must rely on these physicians to render care to their clientele, report significant problems in recruiting and retaining providers. In a number of counties, clients of public programs are experiencing difficulty in obtaining care. Although Medicaid payment rates, traditionally the primary deterrent to physician participation, continue to be a significant drawback, many providers cite malpractice issues as a key reason for not serving low-income patients.

Although the causal relationships among malpractice issues, changes in obstetrical practice, and access to care for low-income women and rural women cannot be precisely documented with the available data, the weight of the evidence is in one direction. *It is reasonable to conclude that access to care for Medicaid and other low-income women is being affected by changes in obstetrical practice generated by professional liability concerns.*

MEDICAID RECIPIENTS AND PROFESSIONAL LIABILITY

Physicians' concerns about professional liability issues can be divided into two categories: (1) the cost of malpractice insurance and (2) the risk of malpractice litigation. Each is an important factor in physicians' practice decisions.

Cost of Insurance Coverage

The rise in malpractice insurance premiums has intensified traditional provider concerns about low rates of Medicaid reimbursement for services. The argument is phrased in two ways. The first contends that payments are too low to cover the costs of malpractice coverage. The second maintains that, in the face of rising malpractice insurance costs, physicians must devote more time to private patients to meet expenses.

It is important to understand that how much a provider *must* charge to meet all expenses, including malpractice insurance, is difficult to ascertain—and depends to some extent on the net income desired by the practitioner. The ACOG reported that in 1986 malpractice premiums represented 20 percent of the average ob-gyn's overhead; the ACOG also reported that premiums represented 10.3 percent of gross income in 1986, compared with 9.7 percent in 1984.[7] Thus, although malpractice premiums rose 46.7 percent in the two years, the proportion of gross income devoted to malpractice insurance rose by only 6.2 percent. This differential must have been covered by increasing charges to private patients.

Because family practitioners tend to have many fewer obstetrical patients than do ob-gyns, for them the higher premiums may pose a clear economic choice. Table 4 uses data from the state of Washington to illustrate this point. Family physicians who do obstetrics paid an additional $9,000 for obstetrical coverage; ob-gyns paid an additional $11,000 above premiums for gynecology only. The family physician performing 30 deliveries a year (the median number) paid $300 per delivery for insurance. Ob-gyns, because of their much larger volumes, had much lower premium costs per delivery. An ob-gyn with the median number of deliveries (121) paid about $93 per delivery for obstetrical malpractice coverage.

Few would disagree that Medicaid programs generally pay providers at rates well below those of private insurers or the average community charge. In 1986 the average Medicaid reimbursement for total obstetrical care rendered by an obstetrician-gynecologist was $550, ranging from $214 to $1,508. Data from 36 states show that Medicaid payments averaged 44 percent of the approximate community charge for prenatal

TABLE 4   Estimated Additional Malpractice Premium Cost Per Delivery, Family Physicians and Obstetrician-Gynecologists in Washington State, 1986

Physician	Number of Deliveries	Added Cost for Malpractice Insurance	Cost of Insurance Per Delivery
Family Physicians			
Median, rural M.D.s	35	9,187	262.49
Median, all M.D.s	30	9,187	306.23
Maximum, rural M.D.s	150	9,187	61.25
Maximum, all M.D.s	200	9,187	45.94
Obstetrician-Gynecologists			
Median, semirural M.D.s	110	11,244	102.22
Median, all M.D.s	121	11,244	92.93
Maximum, semirural M.D.s	210	11,244	53.54
Maximum, all M.D.s	350	11,244	32.13

NOTES: Because no rural ob-gyns were identified, data for specialists in semirural areas were used. The authors reported premiums for family physicians practicing obstetrics at $13,511; premiums for those not practicing obstetrics or performing surgery were $4,324. For ob-gyns, premiums were $33,026 with obstetrics and $21,782 for surgical gynecology without obstetrics.

SOURCE: Rosenblatt, R., and B. Detering. In press. Changing patterns of obstetric practice in Washington State. Family Medicine.

care and routine delivery. The highest state paid 76 percent; the lowest, 14.8 percent.[8] In many cases, these rates represent major increases over prior years because at least 20 states increased payments between 1984 and 1986. Additional increases are being considered—and enacted—by states, particularly those that are adopting the expanded Medicaid coverage options for children and pregnant women available under the Budget Reconciliation Act of 1986.

The problem of low reimbursement rates is complex, reflecting pressures on state budgets, competition among provider types for improved coverage and payments, and general state philosophies regarding Medicaid. The question of whether Medicaid reimbursement *should* reflect the rising costs of malpractice insurance is even more complicated. Should Medicaid reflect the full cost of malpractice coverage? Insurance premiums do not vary with caseload; therefore, one could reasonably argue that service to Medicaid patients is a marginal cost and payments that do not reflect the full cost of coverage are not necessarily unreasonable. If Medicaid reimbursement policies were revised to assume part of the cost of malpractice insurance directly, should these costs include only the obstetrical portion of the premium?

Fear of Litigation

Although insurance costs have been the focus of policy debate, particularly at the state level, risk aversion, or the fear of suit, is an equally strong motivating factor for physicians. Nobody wants to be sued or to have to defend his or her professional abilities in court. Even when the physician wins the case, the psychological impact of having been sued is enormous. Seven out of ten ob-gyns are likely to be sued in the course of their professional lives. Although family physicians are sued less frequently, they may feel more vulnerable because of their less specialized training. The physician's desire to manage his or her individual risk and to avoid situations that might lead to litigation is a normal human response to the current climate.

For low-income women and women covered by Medicaid, access to care may be affected as much—or more—by physicians' fears of suit as by reimbursement rates. As previously noted, low-income patients tend, statistically, to be at greater medical risk; they also tend therefore to be more affected by reductions in the provision of care to high-risk women. In addition it is possible, although difficult to document, that physicians perceive the reduction of care to Medicaid and low-income women as an effective means of reducing their exposure to high-risk patients.

Managing high-risk pregnancies requires a commitment to continuity on the part of patient and physician. If the physician believes that this commitment may not be forthcoming, he or she may be less willing to initiate service. It may be easier for the physician to stop serving Medicaid patients altogether than to attempt to make such judgments (if desired) on an individual basis.

It is ironic that the very factors that call for increased access to care can also intensify a physician's sense of risk when serving low-income patients. The extent to which low-income women receive late or no prenatal care and are therefore at greater risk has been well documented. Indeed, such data are at the heart of the Medicaid expansions recently established by Congress and are the focus of such groups as the National Commission on Infant Mortality Prevention. Yet it is precisely this information that may underlie a physician's sense that service to low-income and Medicaid patients increases the risk of malpractice litigation.

A final issue, which calls for more extensive discussion, is the notion that "the poor sue more." The extent of this belief among physicians is not known, but anecdotal information suggests the belief is held by a significant minority.

This issue raises questions of both phraseology and fact. Does "the poor" refer just to Medicaid recipients or to any low-income person? How is "poor" defined in terms of income? It is possible that the concept of "the poor" is defined by individual perceptions, which could be flawed. The phrase "sue more" could mean that the poor sue more frequently than the rest of the population at risk. Does it mean they bring more "frivolous" suits? If the poor do sue more frequently, is it because they are at greater risk of malpractice incidents than the nonpoor?

To analysts, the statement "the poor sue more" seems almost counterintuitive. The legal literature indicates that the low-income population generally has less access to the legal system—a fact that would lead one to expect the poor to "sue less." Because malpractice actions are frequently brought on a contingent fee basis—and awards are usually based on lost earnings—attorneys should have less financial incentive to take cases for the poor.

Currently available data provide very limited information on the relation of income to malpractice suits. The Department of Health, Education, and Welfare's Commission on Medical Malpractice found in 1973 that greater numbers of "negative medical incidents" were associated with higher incomes (the study did not examine claims rates).[9] A study in Cook County, Illinois, in the 1970s found that black plaintiffs constituted almost 25 percent of the county population but accounted for only 11 percent of malpractice suits.[10] A 1986 study by Weismann and colleagues also found a negative relation between service to minority patients and a physician's likelihood of being sued.[11]

Five studies that specifically examine Medicaid recipients and malpractice litigation arrive at conflicting results.

- Studies of closed claims from malpractice insurers conducted by the U.S. General Accounting Office (GAO)[12] and by the State of Maryland showed that Medicaid recipients brought suit in roughly the same proportion as their numbers in the population. The GAO analyzed a sample of all claims; 5.8 percent were brought by Medicaid patients, who account for about 9 percent of the U.S. population. Average expected payout for a Medicaid plaintiff was almost $25,000; the payout for the average privately insured patient was almost $250,000.[13]
- In Maryland, Medicaid recipients accounted for about 13 percent of ob-gyn service claims between 1977 and 1985. In 1986 Medicaid recipients constituted about 19 percent of obstetrical admissions to Maryland hospitals.[14]
- A nationwide survey of ob-gyns regarding fertility-control services asked several questions about malpractice experience. The study found no significant correlation between Medicaid participation and threatened or actual malpractice litigation.[15]
- Two surveys of providers found higher rates of litigation among Medicaid patients. Respondents in the 1986 Washington State survey of

physicians said that 26 percent of their reported malpractice suits had been initiated by Medicaid recipients, whereas Medicaid patients accounted for only 17.6 percent of their practices. Recently, the ACOG reported on a nationwide survey of hospitals' malpractice claims in 1982. Hospitals reported that Medicaid patients represented 17.1 percent of deliveries but initiated 24.8 percent of malpractice claims (this finding was not statistically significant).[16]

The data that are currently available neither substantiate nor disprove the belief that "the poor sue more." All of the studies suffer from methodological problems that may be inherent in any analysis of this issue.

• Studies of malpractice claims that distinguish among claimants' health insurance status have a very large proportion of claims for which the payer status is unknown. These claims were eliminated in calculating the percentages presented above, a decision that assumes that the unknowns are distributed similarly to the knowns. Given the large number of unknowns, this assumption may be faulty.

• Surveys of physicians are subject to flaws if physicians report perceptions of patient payer status. There is some evidence that physicians tend to overstate the proportion of Medicaid patients in their practice.[17] Study authors in Washington State could not determine whether this type of overstatement affected their data.

• The results of the ACOG hospital survey may have been influenced by the nature of the respondents. One-third of the hospitals had more than 2,000 deliveries—and accounted for 70 percent of the reported claims. In contrast to smaller facilities, hospitals of this size are more likely to be regional neonatal centers or high-risk obstetrical centers—factors that would increase both the Medicaid caseload and the potential for "bad outcomes" and possible malpractice litigation. In addition, large hospitals tend to be in urban areas, which have larger Medicaid populations. Danzon's studies of malpractice have shown that urban areas tend to have higher rates of malpractice litigation generally.[18] Although the total sample drawn by the ACOG was statistically reliable, the size (313 hospitals and 306 claims) does not allow for analysis of differences in claims by hospital size.

CONCLUSIONS

It appears that the professional liability crisis is generating a commensurate crisis in access to maternity services, particularly among low-income women and rural women. If physicians continue to respond to their professional liability concerns by eliminating or reducing their obstetrical services, the access problem is likely to intensify and touch even those areas of the country that are not experiencing problems today. Effective implementation of the new Medicaid expansions will call for creative efforts to address the professional liability concerns of physicians as they relate to participation in Medicaid.

Although the causal relationships between professional liability concerns and service to Medicaid patients are not fully established, Medicaid reimbursement rates and fear of suit appear to be primary factors. The empirical evidence suggesting that physicians who serve Medicaid patients are at greater risk of malpractice litigation is inconclusive at best; yet the perception may have assumed its own reality. In today's litigious climate, the rational response to a belief that service to low-income women increases the risk of litigation is to reduce the provision of such care.

This chapter has focused on the implications of the malpractice insurance crisis for access to obstetrical care. Further research is clearly needed to document trends more fully and to examine the relationship between patient income and malpractice suits; exploration of policy options, however, probably should not await the results of such studies. The weight of current evidence suggests that action may be needed before the research could be completed.

Several states have attempted to address the insurance and access issues. Virginia's new no-fault law includes a requirement that participants in the fund also take part in developing a plan of care for Medicaid recipients and other indigent women. Missouri has adopted provisions to cover liability insurance costs for physicians who contract with local health departments; Montgomery County, Maryland, recently adopted similar provisions.

The federal government could assist states in these endeavors by providing greater flexibility in the Medicaid programs. One route would be to authorize higher Medicaid matching payments in specified situations. In fiscal year 1988 the federal government paid 50 to 80 percent of medical expenditures, with the rate varying among states. States might be eligible for higher matching rates to promote recruitment of physicians in areas with few ob-gyns; to enable the Medicaid program to employ physicians, if necessary; to develop systems of care that might reduce the physician's sense of risk when serving Medicaid recipients; or to experiment with addressing malpractice costs directly by helping to pay premiums.

Another approach would be through defined Medicaid waivers. Medicaid law provides reimbursement for specified services to identified recipients. Under the law, all providers offering that service must be eligible for the same rate, even though payment rates may vary geographically or by specific service. These provisions restrict the ability of states to develop targeted solutions to malpractice-related problems. For example, one state Medicaid program has provided funds to help a local health department in recruiting physicians for health department and Medicaid programs. Other approaches might be to increase reimbursement rates for physicians with large Medicaid practices (to compensate for their rising malpractice insurance costs) or to provide some state funds to pay part of the cost of a malpractice judgment in favor of a Medicaid patient. It appears that these expenditures would not now qualify for federal matching funds.

The U.S. House of Representatives committee report for the budget reconciliation bill of 1987 included a program of Medicaid demonstrations to improve physician participation. As examples of potential demonstrations, the report specifically cited programs to address professional liability concerns, including assistance in paying premiums (or ensuring coverage). The proposal was dropped in the final stages of conference committee negotiation; it may be worth reconsidering.

Further analysis may indicate other ways of easing the access difficulties posed by professional liability concerns. It is important that feasible policy options that address the access issues generated by malpractice concerns be developed and implemented. It would be unfortunate, to say the least, if the national objective of improving maternity care and birth outcomes among low-income women, a goal embodied in the initiatives of the Budget Reconciliation Act of 1986 (and 1987), should founder on the rock of malpractice insurance costs.

REFERENCES AND NOTES

1. Unless otherwise noted, national data on obstetrician-gynecologists are from three American College of Obstetricians and Gynecologists (ACOG) studies: 1983. Professional Liability Insurance and Its Effects: Report of a Survey of ACOG's Membership; 1985. Professional Liability Insurance and Its Effects: Report of a Survey of ACOG's Membership; 1988. Professional Liability and Its Effects: Report of a 1987 Survey of ACOG's Membership. Washington, D.C.
2. Unless otherwise noted, national data on family physicians are from the American Academy of Family Physicians (AAFP). 1986. The Family Physician and Obstetrics: A Professional Liability Study. Kansas City, Mo. The AAFP did a second study, in 1987, but the response rate was much lower than that in the 1986 study.
3. The following state studies (in alphabetical order by state) were reviewed for this report: Alabama Medical Association. 1985. State of Alabama Survey on Obstetrical Care; Crump, W., and D. Redmond. 1986. Final report: A survey of family physicians providing OB care. Ala. Med.; Darnell, H. 1986. Current status of family practice obstetrics in Alabama. Ala. Med. (September):36–38; Gordon, R. J., G. McMullen, B. D. Weiss, and A. W. Nichols. 1987. The effect of malpractice liability on the delivery

of rural obstetrical care. J. Rural Health (Arizona) 3:7–13; California Academy of Family Physicians. 1985. Rural hospital center survey. Memorandum. December 6; California Medical Association. 1987. Professional liability issues in obstetrical practice. Socioecon. Rep. 25, nos. 6 and 7; Medical Society of the District of Columbia. 1985. Survey of obstetricians; Georgia Obstetrical and Gynecological Society. 1985 and 1987. Manpower surveys; Idaho Medical Association. 1987. Survey of members; Illinois Department of Public Health. 1987. Changes in Availability of Obstetrical Services in Illinois; Iowa Medical Society and Iowa Academy of Family Physicians. 1985. Survey of family physicians; Kansas Medical Society. 1985. Professional liability survey. Kans. Med. 43; Bonham, G. S. 1987. Survey of Kentucky obstetrical practice. University of Louisville, Urban Studies Center, Louisville; Ob/Gyn Society of Maryland. 1986. Survey; Weissman, C., M. Teitelbaum, and D. Celentana. 1987. Physicians' practice changes in response to malpractice litigation. Paper presented at the American Public Health Association annual meeting, October 20 (Maryland); Massachusetts Ob-Gyn Society. 1986. Survey; Block, M. 1985. Professional Liability Insurance and Obstetrical Practice. Study commissioned by the Michigan State Medical Society and the American College of Obstetricians and Gynecologists. Lansing; Minnesota Ob-Gyn Liaison Committee. 1986. Survey; Smucker, D. R. 1988. Obstetrics in family practice in the state of Ohio. J. Fam. Prac. 26:165–168; Oregon Medical Association. 1987. The Impact of Malpractice Issues on Patient Care: Declining Availability of Obstetrical Services in Oregon. Portland; Texas Medical Association. 1985 and 1986. Professional liability insurance surveys; Virginia Obstetrical and Gynecological Society. 1985. Survey of Virginia ob-gyns; University of Washington School of Public Health and Community Medicine. 1986. The Effects of Changes in the Medical Liability Market on Washington Obstetricians. Final Report to the Washington State Medical Association. Seattle; Rosenblatt, R. A., and B. Detering. In press. Changing patterns of obstetric practice in Washington State. Fam. Med.; Rosenblatt, R. A., and C. L. Wright. 1987. Rising malpractice premiums and obstetric practice patterns. Western J. Med. 146:246–248; West Virginia State Medical Association. 1985. Physician survey.

4. In addition to the three ACOG studies and the two AAFP surveys cited above, national studies include Tietze, P. E., P. S. Gaskins, and M. McGinnis. 1988. Attrition from obstetrical practice among family practice residency graduates. J. Fam. Prac. 26:204–205; MACRO Systems, Inc. 1986. Medical Malpractice Liability Coverage in the 1980s: Threat to Patient Access to Health Care? Final Report. Washington, D.C.; National Governors' Association, Center for Policy Research, Health Policy Studies. 1988. Increasing Provider Participation: Strategies for Improving State Perinatal Care Programs. Washington, D.C.; Weissman, C., M. Teitelbaum, and L. Morlock. 1988. Malpractice claims experience associated with fertility-control services among young obstetrician-gynecologists. Med. Care 26:298–306.

5. State of Colorado, Department of Social Services, fiscal year 1989 budget hearings.

6. National Governors' Association. 1988; see note 4.

7. ACOG. 1988, p. 12.

8. National Governors' Association. 1988; see note 4. The report includes discussion of the methodology used in developing the estimates.

9. U.S. Department of Health, Education, and Welfare. 1973. Report of the Secretary's Commission on Medical Malpractice. DHEW Pub. no. (OS) 73-89. Washington, D.C.: Government Printing Office, pp. 658–694. These data do not mean that the poor experience fewer incidents of malpractice; rather, the author hypothesized that the poor may be less likely to perceive an experience as a case of malpractice.

10. National Health Law Program. 1987. Medical Malpractice: A "Crisis" for Poor Women. Clearinghouse Review. Los Angeles, pp. 1277–1286.
11. Weissman et al. 1988; see note 4.
12. General Accounting Office (GAO), U.S. Congress. 1987. Medical Malpractice: Characteristics of Claims Closed in 1984. GAO/HRD-87-55. Gaithersburg, Md.
13. Retabulation of the GAO data was provided by Laura Morlock, The Johns Hopkins University. The published GAO data include payout in one year. Morlock retabulated the data to include total payout over time.
14. Unpublished data on 10 years of malpractice claims were provided by Laura Morlock, The Johns Hopkins University. Hospital admission data were provided by the Maryland Health Services Cost Review Commission.
15. Weissman et al. 1988; see note 4.
16. American College of Obstetricians and Gynecologists. 1988. Hospital Survey on Obstetric Claim Frequency by Patient Payor Category. Washington, D.C.
17. Kletke, P. R., S. M. Davidson, J. D. Perloff, D. W. Schiff, and J. P. Connelly. 1985. The extent of physician participation in Medicaid: A comparison of physician estimates and aggregated patient records. Health Serv. Res. 20:503–523.
18. Danzon, P. 1986. The frequency and severity of medical malpractice claims: New evidence. Law Contemp. Prob. 49(Spring):57–84.

Medical Professional Liability and the Relations Between Doctors and Their Patients

ARNOLD RELMAN, M.D.

In my judgment, the problem of medical malpractice liability has four root causes. I believe they are all important, and I mention them in no special order.

CAUSES OF THE PROBLEM

Malpractice

The first of these root causes is malpractice itself. However uncomfortable it makes us feel, we physicians must recognize that there are incompetent and impaired physicians who ought not to be practicing medicine and who are prone to errors that may do serious harm to patients. They probably constitute a tiny faction of the profession, but nobody knows exactly how many there are. In any case, they often manage to escape detection and disciplining by peer review state licensing bodies, at least for a long time, and they probably account for a large share of malpractice actions. A variant of this problem is the otherwise competent physician who is doing something for which he or she has not been adequately trained and who therefore performs ineptly.

Although there are no data on this point, I would guess that the great majority of physician defendants in malpractice actions would be judged by their peers to be generally competent and unimpaired, and qualified to provide the service that preceded the plaintiff's injury. Furthermore, I suspect that qualified and unbiased experts with access to all of the

97

relevant facts would find only a small fraction of cases in which the care provided by the physician had been inept. Unfortunately, there is no reliable evidence on this score, but I think it is safe to say that malpractice is by no means the only cause and probably not even the major cause of malpractice actions.

The Tort System

A second explanation for the rising tide of malpractice actions is to be found in the perverse incentives inherent in the present tort system. The contingency fee arrangement encourages patients to take legal action. It also gives lawyers a powerful reason to seek out plaintiffs and to ask juries for large settlements. The outcome of the adversarial courtroom drama, played before a lay jury, is often influenced more by emotion, legal histrionics, and the testimony of hired-gun "expert" witnesses than by the weight of scientific evidence and the opinion of unbiased authorities. Huge awards for "pain and suffering" are common and tend to drive up costs.

The most perverse aspect of the whole system is its failure to provide for compensation without proving malpractice. Maloccurrence, which justifies compensation, does not necessarily mean that malpractice has occurred. At present, however, compensation for iatrogenic injuries depends on convincing a jury that there has been malpractice by the physician (or the hospital). The system, in other words, forces all patients seeking compensation for an injury to convince a jury that some person or institution is at fault, even though frequently there is reasonable doubt about such fault.

The fact that most malpractice cases are decided in favor of the defendant suggests that legal action is very often initiated without sufficient evidence to support the claim. Nevertheless, this circumstance does not mean that the plaintiff has not suffered injury at the hands of the medical care system nor that the plaintiff is undeserving of compensation. The basic problem here is that there is no way for the plaintiff to get that compensation without taking legal action against the health care provider. This basic distortion of logic must ultimately be corrected if we are ever to solve the malpractice problem.

Social Attitudes

The epidemic of malpractice litigation is due also to a general change in social attitudes. We live in an increasingly litigious society in which there is a growing tendency to assign personal responsibility for almost every misfortune and to use the legal system to gain compensation from those believed to be at fault. Liability actions are increasing in many sectors, not just in medicine, and liability insurance costs for many private businesses and public institutions are rising rapidly. The growth of a more militant consumerism adds to the pressure for litigation, as does a growing public skepticism about the medical profession. Physicians in general no longer have the unquestioned public trust and esteem they enjoyed a generation ago. The image of the doctor as omniscient and beneficent has been tarnished by a spate of stories in the media about incompetent, venal, and unethical physicians and by a growing suspicion of all authority.

Commercialization of Medicine

The commercialization of medicine, which has become increasingly apparent during the past 10 or 15 years, contributes to this erosion of public trust. The growing tendency of hospitals and other health care institutions to act like businesses—and of many physicians to act like businessmen—has changed the attitudes of patients. When the Samaritan ethic was more in evidence and patients believed that their doctors were more interested in their welfare than in economic gain, liability actions were unlikely, even when things went very wrong. But when medical care becomes primarily a commercial transaction and patients are treated as customers, the climate changes.

As customers, patients are more inclined to demand total satisfaction and to seek legal redress when the results of their medical care are disappointing. Litigation, after all, is a frequent resort when relations between the parties in a commercial transaction become troubled. It ought to be only rarely used in a properly functioning doctor-patient relationship because patients who see their physicians as trusted counselors rather than as vendors of services demand only that they be competent and caring. Patients who trust their doctors and believe they are doing their best are more philosophical about disappointing outcomes.

EFFECTS OF THE MALPRACTICE CRISIS ON DOCTOR-PATIENT RELATIONS

These general considerations bring me to a consideration of the main topic of this discussion: how relations between doctors and patients affect, and are affected by, the malpractice crisis. There is no doubt that among the major causes of this crisis are the attitudes doctors and patients have toward each other and the way doctors and patients interact. Equally certain is that concern about malpractice litigation has powerful effects, both good and bad, on the practice behavior of many physicians. In focusing on these aspects of the subject I do not wish to minimize the importance of the others mentioned above. No satisfactory solution of the malpractice dilemma is likely to be achieved without attention to all of the causes I have outlined, but I have been asked to limit my comments to this part of the problem. In a symposium as wide-ranging as this one, the subject of doctor-patient relations obviously needs close attention.

As an internist, I am not qualified to discuss the special problems of obstetrical practice. Most of my comments will be of a general nature, and to the extent that they are valid, they apply to obstetrical care as well as to other areas of medical practice. I must also point out that, because the literature has almost no factual evidence bearing on this subject, I am reduced simply to expressing my opinions, which are based on reasonably extensive clinical experience. Although I believe my views will be supported by most experienced physicians, they nevertheless must be acknowledged to be opinions.

With those caveats, let me begin by considering how the attitudes of patients and doctors and the practice style of doctors affect the likelihood of a malpractice action.

Changes in Attitudes

The first thing that must be said is that a patient is much less likely to sue a physician if they know each other well, if the patient trusts the physician, and if the physician tells the patient whatever he or she would like to know, explaining as much as possible and honestly facing up to any failures in diagnosis or treatment.

When most physicians were primary care givers, personal contact between doctor and patient was maximized. The decline in the dominance of primary care practice and the increasing prevalence of specialists have reduced the patient's personal contact with the doctor. Many specialists are virtual strangers to their patients.

Specialization also means the introduction of many new technical procedures, which not only gives rise to greater expectations by patients but also increases the risks of incompetence and expands the possibility of malpractice. Specialized technology makes it possible to do more for patients, but it also tends to estrange doctors and patients. It is hardly surprising that, when anything goes wrong, specialists are more likely to be sued than primary care physicians. It is for this reason that the malpractice premium rates for specialists, who perform technical procedures, are higher than for general physicians, who primarily offer counsel and relatively simple office procedures.

Changes in Practice Organization

The rise of group practice might affect malpractice risk in different directions. On the one hand, physicians in groups are more likely to be under close, continuous peer review and less likely than those in solo practice to be impaired or incompetent. This factor would suggest that bad outcomes leading to malpractice actions might be less common. On the other hand, physicians in group practice are more likely to share responsibility for their patients and therefore to be less closely bonded to them. For example, in large group obstetrical practices whose physicians rotate being on call, it is common for a woman to be assisted with her delivery by an obstetrician who has not provided most of her prenatal care. This factor might suggest a greater likelihood of patient dissatisfaction. I do not know the net effect of group practice on liability. Do physicians in group practice experience the same rate of malpractice actions as their colleagues in solo or partnership practice? I have been told that the costs of liability coverage in some groups are about one-third less than those of solo practitioners in the same community, but I do not know of any published information on this point. It would be interesting to have such data.

At this juncture I need to say something about "informed consent." Informed consent is a popular concept these days—but more a concept than reality because it is rarely possible to inform a patient fully about all the possible consequences of a proposed procedure. Furthermore, the urgency of the medical circumstances often gives the patient (or his or her surrogate) little choice but to sign a consent form. In addition, although informed consent documents are routinely used for surgical and invasive diagnostic procedures, it is impractical to use them for all of the vast array of diagnostic and nonsurgical therapeutic procedures employed in the everyday practice of ambulatory and inpatient medicine. In any case informed consent does not immunize physicians against legal action by patients who claim to have been injured by the incompetent practice of medicine, although it probably lessens the risk.

Changes in Physician Behavior

So far, I have been describing how the attitudes of doctors and patients and the organization of medical practice can affect the likelihood of malpractice actions. I would now like to consider how the growing threat of litigation can, in turn, influence the behavior of doctors. Those who believe that the threat of litigation is necessary to keep physicians aware of their professional responsibilities and that it may have salutary effects on medical practice have some reason on their side. Many physicians have undoubtedly become more cautious and more concerned to see that nothing is overlooked in their care of patients. In obstetrical practice, more attention is probably being paid to all of the details of prenatal care. Counseling, explanation, and informed consent are emphasized more, and obstetricians probably take greater pains to discuss all of the options for prenatal diagnosis. In general, physicians who worry about the threat of litigation are more likely to document everything they do very carefully and to seek consultation more readily when they are in doubt about a diagnosis or treatment. All of this is to the good.

Yet the increasingly litigious climate has many negative effects as well. If physicians have become more cautious, they have also become more suspicious and defensive toward their patients. Patients are likely to be seen as potential courtroom adversaries, thus straining the traditional bonds of beneficent concern and good will. If doctors are now more motivated to ensure careful, detailed workups of their patients, they are also often intimidated by the threat of litigation and as a result are more likely to do too much. One often sees physicians ordering tests and consultations simply to protect themselves against possible subsequent legal action, even when the tests are redundant and unnecessary. This practice, of course, increases the cost and risk of medical care. In obstetrics, the growing—and probably excessive—use of fetal monitoring and cesarean sections undoubtedly stems in part from this fear of the legal action that might result should the pregnancy yield anything less than a perfect baby.

Much has been said about the national cost of this kind of "defensive medicine," as it occurs in all types of practice. Some observers consider this trend to be a major factor in the overall inflation of medical costs, but there are no reliable data on this point. Certainly, the cost must be considerable, particularly if the secondary consequences of the excessive diagnostic studies, such as the additional testing generated by false-positive results and the morbidity of the procedures, are included.

Defensive medicine can also lead physicians to withdraw their services. In some of the high-risk surgical specialties, such as orthopedics, neurosurgery, and obstetrics, physicians have been retiring early or changing their practices to avoid seeing patients with clinical problems that carry a high likelihood of malpractice litigation. In some areas of the country this stance has led to shortages of tertiary care specialists and obstetricians. Exorbitant liability insurance premiums in high-risk specialties and fear of involvement in malpractice suits are undoubtedly discouraging many physicians from entering or staying in these specialties, but the exact extent of the problem and the role of other factors have not been clarified.

Even the increased attention given to informing patients more fully about alternatives and consequences—which helps to avoid misunderstandings and false expectations—has its negative side. Some physicians, particularly those with relatively little experience, are so eager to avoid responsibility that they abdicate their role as trustee and counsellor. They lay out all the possibilities and choices and leave the decisions to the patient. Some patients clearly want to be in that position, and for them such behavior is fine; but most patients, after a modest amount of explanation from their physician, want him or her to take the lead in recommending a course of action. They need reassurance. They want to feel that their doctor is shouldering most of the responsibility and the worry and will stand by them, no matter what happens. On far too many occasions I have seen physicians act simply as technicians, providing the medical services patients seek but not the counsel and support they also need.

I believe this abdication of professional responsibility reflects many currents in our culture, but surely one of its major causes is the growing wariness many physicians feel as they think about the possibility of malpractice action in the event of any untoward outcome of their work.

SUMMARY

I have emphasized that an important source of the malpractice problem is the changed relationship between doctor and patient, which results from the rise of specialization, the commercialization of medical practice, and the erosion of the physician's public image. At the same time, a growing awareness of the malpractice threat is changing the way physicians treat patients—in ways both salutary and deleterious but on balance probably damaging to the practice of medicine. The malpractice problem is complex, deep-seated, and pervasive. It is not likely to be solved by anything less than a fundamentally new approach to the compensation of iatrogenic injuries and a determined effort by the medical profession to deal with the root causes of public dissatisfaction.

Professional Liability Insurance and Nurse-Midwifery Practice

SARAH D. COHN, C.N.M., J.D.

A certified nurse-midwife is an individual educated in the two disciplines of nursing and midwifery and certified according to the requirements of the American College of Nurse-Midwives (ACNM). Nurse-midwifery practice is the independent management of the care of essentially normal newborns and women antepartally, intrapartally, postpartally, and gynecologically within a health care system that provides for medical consultation, collaborative management, or referral and is in accord with the functions, standards, and qualifications for nurse-midwifery practice as defined by the ACNM.[1]

The American College of Nurse-Midwives was incorporated in 1955 in New Mexico and functions as a trade association for nurse-midwives in the United States. In the early 1970s the college began to certify nurse-midwives for beginning competency—that is, certification took place after completion of an approved educational program of study; the certificate was not renewable. At the time the examination of graduating students was begun, a mechanism was created for retroactively certifying nurse-midwives already in practice. The ACNM has certified approximately 3,900 nurse-midwives since then. Of these, approximately 2,500 are members of ACNM (the number is higher if student members are included).

Nurse-midwives differ from so-called lay midwives in several respects. Training is the first difference: nurse-midwives must complete an approved educational program, and candidates for certification may not take the certification examination unless their program director affirms that they have completed basic preparation. The ACNM maintains a set of core competencies and approves educational programs. Training for lay midwives is not standardized. Background is the second difference: nurse-midwives must have a current R.N. (registered nurse) license from a jurisdiction in the United States at the time they take the certification examination. The states in which nurse-midwifery is practiced may also require an active nursing license; in fact the majority of states regulate nurse-midwifery practice as part of nurse-practitioner regulation. Although many lay midwives are also nurses, nursing qualifications are not a requirement for practice, even in those states that regulate lay midwives.

A third difference is the requirement for physician collaboration: nurse-midwives are required (by the ACNM and many states) to maintain a collaborative relationship or practice agreement with a qualified physician who can provide service to patients if needed. This requirement does not mean that the nurse-midwife must be employed by a physician or that the physician must be on the premises to supervise, but it does mean that the nurse-midwife must have made necessary referral arrangements. Lay midwives have long found it difficult to arrange qualified medical backup, and some of them practice without it, using the local emergency room as the referral site. A fourth difference is in scope of practice: as the definition of nurse-midwifery makes clear, nurse-midwives provide prenatal, delivery, and gynecological care to women and initial care to infants. Lay midwives may provide some prenatal care and perform deliveries, but they do not provide follow-up care. Deliveries by lay midwives invariably take place outside the hospital; nurse-midwives deliver babies both in and out of hospitals, depending on the practice.

Nurse-midwives serve thousands of women and families across the country. The ACNM sponsors a study of nurse-midwifery practice approximately every five years. Surveys from 1976–1977 and 1982 have been published by the ACNM; data from the 1987 study have been collected and are being tabulated. As of 1982, the ACNM had certified 2,550 nurse-midwives; 1,684 responded to the survey.[2] Respondents reported that they were practicing in every state but Indiana[3] and were performing deliveries in every state but Idaho, Indiana, and North Dakota. Fourteen percent performed home deliveries; an additional 12 percent performed deliveries in nonhospital birth centers. Respondents reported 68,165 deliveries, or 1.8 percent of all deliveries in the United States during 1982.[4]

Some of the data on patient characteristics are already available from the survey (Table 1). They show that nurse-midwives' patients tend to be slightly older, of lower parity, and somewhat better educated than the total population of childbearing women. One exception is the disproportionate number of women under age 15: nurse-midwives delivered four times as many women under age 15 as their general distribution in the population of providers would suggest. These data should be examined in light of practice requirements: nurse-midwives generally treat low-risk patients and are unlikely to manage patients with hypertension, a very low hematocrit, or gestations of more than 42 weeks without physician consultation.[5] Nurse-midwives working in the region comprising Arizona, Nevada, New Mexico, and Utah conducted the highest mean number of deliveries per year.[6]

The ACNM does not collect data on the number or percentage of patients for whom care is reimbursed by Medicaid.

TABLE 1   Mothers Whose Babies Were Delivered by Nurse-Midwives (N-Ms) in the 12 Months Prior to the 1982 American College of Nurse Midwives (ACNM) Survey and All Mothers Who Delivered in the United States in 1977, by Age, Parity, and Education

Maternal Characteristic	Percent Distribution of Deliveries by N-Ms[a]	Percent Distribution of All Deliveries[b]
Age	(283 Reporting practices)	
Under 15	1.2	0.3
15–19	15.3	16.8
20–29	59.0	65.0
30–39	22.6	17.1
40 +	1.9	0.8
Total	100.0	100.0
Parity	(274 Reporting practices)	
One	45.1	42.1
Two or three	43.5	47.2
Four or more	11.4	10.7
Total	100.0	100.0
Education	(215 Reporting practices)	
Less than high school	18.1	26.2
Completion of high school	30.2	44.9
More than high school	20.6	16.3
College degree or more	31.1	12.6
Total	100.0	100.0

[a]Data reported by directors of nurse-midwifery practices who were U.S. residents and respondents in the ACNM survey, Nurse-Midwifery in the United States: 1982 (Washington, D.C., 1984).

[b]Calculated from data published in Vital Statistics of the United States, 1977. Vol. 1, Natality. DHHS Pub. no. (PHS) 81-1113 (Hyattsville, Md., 1981).

PROFESSIONAL LIABILITY INSURANCE FOR NURSE-MIDWIVES

In the 1982 survey only 47 respondents, or 4.4 percent, did not carry professional liability insurance.[7] Of these, 24 (51.1 percent) were working in the U.S. military and thus were covered under the Federal Tort Claims Act. This act permits malpractice claims to be brought, but the defendant must be the United States; the plaintiff may not name individual defendants. More than half (53 percent) of the 1,018 nurse-midwives who gave information on their insurance coverage stated that they carried a personal policy only; 31 percent carried a personal policy and were also insured by an employer's policy.

The ACNM began offering a professional liability insurance policy for its members in 1974. In 1976 approximately 625 nurse-midwives were insured. By 1983 the number of insured had risen to 1,400; by late 1984 it had reached 2,400. The individual premium was less than $250 in 1983.[8] Between 1977 and 1982, ACNM members paid more than $230,000 in premiums; during the same period, the insurer paid losses or accumulated reserves on open cases totaling $1.1 million. In 1984, with a new insurance carrier, premiums began to rise rapidly for nurse-midwives, whose mean annual income was $22,982.[9] Between 1974 and 1984, the ACNM professional liability insurance offered was occurrence based.[10] Beginning in 1981, $1 million per claim protection was available for purchase.

In 1984 the commercial carrier that was insuring nurse-midwives canceled the master policy. The ACNM found another commercial carrier, but policies with that company were canceled within a year. At the time these policies were canceled, about 1,400 nurse-midwives were insured.[11] The last company has become insolvent and is now administered by a trustee. During 1984 and 1985, the ACNM began to explore three options for ACNM-sponsored professional liability insurance. First, it continued to try to find a suitable commercial carrier, as this was the option that seemed the most responsive to membership needs. Second, it considered setting up a captive insurance company in a suitable U.S. or foreign jurisdiction. Finally, it considered the possibility of being unable to offer any policy. At the same time, the federal legislation that became the Risk Retention Act was proposed and supported by the ACNM.

In July 1986, after approximately one year without an ACNM-sponsored professional liability insurance policy, the ACNM membership was offered a commercial policy by a consortium of insurers led by CNA Insurance Company. The maximum amount of insurance a nurse-midwife can buy is $1 million per claim/$1 million annual aggregate. The policy is of the claims-made type;[12] a reporting endorsement[13] will be payable for any nurse-midwife who leaves the company and does not have other coverage. The insurance consortium agreed to offer the insurance for at least several years to avoid the problem of a cancelation after one or two years, with the resulting reporting endorsement payment for every insured if no subsequent company offered prior acts coverage.[14]

As with commercial claims-made insurance offered to physicians, premiums under the ACNM policy rise for five years until the policy is considered mature. The maximum policy costs approximately $6,000 per year. In contrast to physician policies, there is no gynecology-only rate; nurse-midwives who choose this insurance pay the same premium whether or not they are performing deliveries. Also in contrast to physicians' insurance, the cost of the policy is the same in every state, and the consortium does not offer a rate for part-time practice.

The 1982 survey data show that only 55 nurse-midwives (5.2 percent) had ever been sued.[15] This low rate is in sharp contrast to the 70 percent of obstetricians reporting suits in the latest survey by the American College of Obstetricians and Gynecologists (ACOG).[16] The ACNM claims data (which include information only from policies handled by the ACNM-sponsored insurer and not from other commercial policies) were analyzed by actuaries when ACNM was examining the possibility of sponsoring an insurance company. Their reports indicated that the claims rate and severity data were insufficient for setting premiums. Some actuaries have used these same data to project very high premiums for nurse-midwives; the justification for this practice appears to be that when data are insufficient, nurse-midwifery risk is rated at a percentage of obstetrician risk. That percentage in turn can be an estimate that may be inflated to protect the insurer from unanticipated losses.

These professional liability insurance problems have affected the practice of nurse-midwifery, its structure and integrity, and job opportunities for nurse-midwives. They have also created difficulties for nurse-midwives in obtaining hospital privileges and have increased the costs of nurse-midwifery services to patients.

Effects on Structure of Practice

In 1985 when the ACNM master policy was canceled for the final time, many groups of professionals were having liability problems. The ACOG master policy was canceled at about the same time; however, physicians could still obtain insurance in the states in which they practiced, albeit often at high rates. For nurse-midwives the situation was different. For example, in Connecticut, then and now, there are three commercial carriers that insure obstetricians; none of these carriers will insure a nurse-midwife who is not employed by a physician insured with the company. This requirement forced out of business two nurse-midwifery practices that had hired physicians to provide medical coverage for them when needed. When the nurse-midwives were unable to buy professional liability insurance at any price except as employees, the practices were closed.

A nurse-midwifery practice that employs physicians rather than vice versa is considered by some to be innovative and desirable. Yet without insurance, practice, although not legally prohibited (most states do not require health care professionals to be insured), is practically impossible. Nonhospital birth centers, another innovation in care, were drastically affected by the loss of both their own policies (institutional) and the ACNM master policy; those centers that survived generally rely on their professionals to find and carry professional liability coverage.

Now that commercial insurance is again available to nurse-midwives through a consortium, it is tempting to believe that practices can continue to develop. Hospitals, however, generally require that their non-employed professional and medical staffs carry professional liability insurance; when a minimum amount is specified, it is usually $1 million per claim/$3 million annual aggregate. At this time, the consortium does not offer insurance to nurse-midwives in excess of $1 million per claim/$1 million annual aggregate, an amount that is insufficient to satisfy many hospitals. Hospitals will therefore deny privileges unless the nurse-midwife can find other insurance.

Nurse-midwives in some states have been successful in seeking to be insured by the state joint underwriting authority. Premiums for this coverage vary from state to state.

Effects of Insurance Surcharges

Some liability carriers have imposed premium surcharges on physicians who employ or work with nurse-midwives. Data collected by the ACOG in 1987 showed that 7.7 percent of the 1,648 respondents employed nurse-midwives in full- or part-time staff positions; 19.5 percent employed nurse-practitioners. Of the 127 who employed nurse-midwives, 47 percent had had a professional liability surcharge imposed.[17]

An ACNM survey of nurse-midwives found that approximately 10 percent of physicians associated with nurse-midwifery practices had experienced surcharges.[18] Of the 1,229 nurse-midwives responding, 899 were in clinical practice; 78 of them reported that their practices had been affected by physician surcharges, and 13 reported that their practices had been closed. Twenty-five insurance companies were named by the nurse-midwives, many of them physician owned. The amounts charged ranged from $94 to $23,000 per physician annually.[19]

Changes in Practice

In May 1988 two nurse-midwifery students reported on a study they had done on the effects on nurse-midwifery practice of changes in professional liability insurance costs and coverage.[20] Data from the 300 questionnaires that were returned and analyzed indicated that the average insurance premium amount of $4,000 was about 14 percent of a nurse-midwife's gross income. Sixty-four percent of nurse-midwives were working full time; 21 percent were working part time. In 78 percent of the practices the employer paid the insurance premium; in 16 percent nurse-midwives paid their own; and in 6 percent they split the costs. Seventy-two percent of the respondents had increased their patient-care fees the preceding year; the average cost of prenatal care and delivery was $1,300 per client. The study noted that, although health insurance premiums had risen 114 percent between 1984 and 1988, nurse-midwifery fees had risen 18 percent and nurse-midwifery income had risen 7 percent.

Respondents were asked about the effects of insurance costs on their techniques of practice. Twenty-one percent stated that they were ordering more diagnostic ultrasound testing; 20 percent said they were doing more nonstress testing; 19 percent reported more laboratory testing; and 16 percent said they were doing more electronic fetal monitoring. Thirteen percent of the nurse-midwives responding were giving up nurse-midwifery practice: 34 percent of them cited the increased cost of coverage and 6 percent cited the decreased amount of coverage as the reasons. In answer to another question, more than 30 percent of nurse-midwives indicated that there were fewer job opportunities than there had been before the costs of insurance rose and coverage decreased.

The study was not extensive enough to determine trends in the availability of nurse-midwifery services to Medicaid patients; for example, the survey questions regarding fee for service did not produce the detailed information needed to trace such trends.

CONCLUSION

For the average nurse-midwife, who earns a gross salary of $30,000 per year and pays $5,000 for professional liability insurance off the top, there may not be enough money left to adequately pay other practice and living expenses. Although an obstetrician's premium averages 10 percent of his or her annual gross income,[21] that gross income averages $296,000.[22] Nurse-midwives whose physician-employers pay their professional liability insurance premiums are under pressure to earn their salary plus the insurance expense; this is an economic fact of life, but it may have the effect of decreasing job opportunities for nurse-midwives. Unless nurse-midwives find a way to balance insurance premiums and salaries, it will be difficult for those who are so inclined to establish practices in more remote areas of the country and among poorer patients.

REFERENCES AND NOTES

1. These two definitions were accepted by the board of directors of the American College of Nurse-Midwives in January 1978.
2. American College of Nurse Midwives (ACNM). 1984. Nurse-Midwifery in the United States: 1982. Washington, D.C., p. 1.
3. Ibid., p. 25.
4. Ibid., p. 39.
5. Ibid., p. 50.
6. Ibid., p. 40.
7. Ibid., p. 37.
8. Cohn, S. 1984. The nurse-midwife: Malpractice and risk management. J. Nurse-Midwifery 29:316–321.
9. ACNM. 1984; see note 2.
10. For an annual premium, the insurance company will insure professional liability claims made or suits brought involving incidents that occurred during the policy year, no matter how many years have elapsed when the claim is made.
11. ACNM testimony before the Senate Committee on Commerce, Science, and Transportation, March 4, 1986, p. 4.
12. For an annual premium, the insurance company will insure professional liability claims brought during the policy year, as long as the incident also occurred during that year or during a prior year in which the same company provided insurance. The annual policy will not cover claims brought in a later year if there is no policy active with the same company (and no reporting endorsement or prior acts coverage—see notes 13 and 14).
13. A reporting endorsement insures claims brought after the expiration of a claims-made policy; it is usually a one-time premium to provide so-called tail coverage for the prior year or years covered by a claims-made policy.
14. An insured person who moves from one professional liability carrier to another, both operating under a claims-made format, may obtain from the new company reporting endorsement coverage for claims brought on earlier incidents. This is called prior acts coverage.
15. ACNM. 1984; see note 2.
16. American College of Obstetricians and Gynecologists (ACOG). 1988. Professional Liability and Its Effects: Report of a 1987 Survey of ACOG's Membership. Washington, D.C., Table 18.
17. Ibid., Tables 11 and 12.
18. Data reported verbally by Gail Sinquefeld at the 33rd ACNM annual convention, Detroit, Michigan, May 1988.

19. Ibid.
20. Patch, F. B., and S. Holaday. 1988. Effects of changes to professional liability insurance and certified nurse-midwives. Paper presented at the American College of Nurse-Midwives 33rd annual convention research forum. Detroit, Michigan.
21. ACOG. 1988, Table 16; see note 16.
22. Ibid.

The Legal Issues

Market and Regulatory Approaches to Medical Malpractice: The Virginia Obstetrical No-Fault Statute

RICHARD A. EPSTEIN, LL.B.

The question of medical malpractice and its legal consequences has long been of concern to lawyers and physicians. For years, however, it seemed to be a problem that was well under control, given the array of doctrines and practices that has grown up around it. Today, medical care on average is probably better and more sophisticated than it has ever been before. Yet since roughly 1975,[1] the medical profession has regarded itself as under siege by a set of legal developments that both lawyers and judges have defended as merely the regular and traditional application of the ordinary rules of civil responsibility to physicians, who are, after all, no more special than anyone else.

Everyone cannot be right, but everyone can be wrong. With respect to medical malpractice, I think this second possibility is too close to the truth. There are essentially two general questions that must be decided in fashioning any system of medical malpractice responsibility. First, who should decide the applicable norms for a given transaction? Second, what should those norms be? The traditional view of the subject has been that the first of these questions is easy to answer, whereas the second is more difficult. On the initial question of the allocation of power, the applicable standards should be set up either by courts or by legislatures, under a system in which the latter can override the judgment of the former unless and until the constitutional rights of individual patients are infringed. With the locus of power thus established, the debate then switches to the choice of collective standards that are applicable across the board. What are the rules for informed consent, for setting the standard of care, for proving breach of duty, for measuring damages, or for taking collateral sources of compensation into account? The number of permutations within the framework of a tort medical malpractice system is legion. The set of possibilities is augmented yet again by more radical proposals that jettison the "fault" standard and proceed on wholly different fault principles.[2] Generally, obstetrics and gynecology are not regarded as requiring special rules—and justifiably so. The Virginia Birth-Related Neurological Injury Compensation Act (Injured Infant Act),[3] which is discussed in greater detail later in this chapter, applies only to a limited class of obstetrical injuries and is therefore a clear, and ominous, exception to the general approach.

The common mistake of the modern system of medical malpractice responsibility is its facile answer to the first question. Why is it assumed that some outside collective body—court or legislature—should have the last word on the design of systems to deal with medical malpractice or medical maloccurrences? The rival system of private contracts between patients and physicians, who can then decide these questions for themselves, is typically given very short shrift.[4] Yet once this possibility is taken more seriously, the pressure for unanimous or substantial agreement on the substantive issues is removed. If physician A and patient B structure their arrangements one way, physician C and patient D are free to imitate them or to disregard that arrangement if they choose. The dominant question is no longer what single set of rules shall govern all transactions but who shall decide which rules are applicable in any individual case. The first function of legislatures is to make clear that ordinary freedoms to contract may be exercised. The function of courts is reduced to the modest one of enforcing contracts as drafted. Thereafter, the legislature should simply stay its hand.

This last condition of legislative inaction explains why it will be so difficult to implement contract solutions: markets always operate at the mercy of legislative intervention. Moreover, there is today sustained and decisive political objection to any return to a marketplace for medical goods and services. Putting aside, for a moment, these practical political objections, I think that it is possible to find reasons why a system of contracts and markets works for most goods and services. This general solution can then be extended to the specific problems of obstetrical care.

THE LOGIC OF MARKETS: WHY CONTRACT?

The basic logic of contracting is simple and appealing. Everyone generally starts with individual endowments in wealth, intelligence, and skills. Physicians have their labor; hospitals, their resources; and patients, their wealth and natural talents. (For these purposes at least, we can put aside the question of how anyone comes by any particular entitlement in the first place.) Contracting parties also have a certain measure of self-interest, but that self-interest should not be too narrowly defined; parents, for example, have a deep concern for the welfare of their children and will generally contract on their behalf. All parties are allowed to exchange their endowments for others they do not possess. The exchanges can take place on whatever terms they see fit. Force and misrepresentation, however, as well as contracting with infants and incompetents, are ruled out as improper forms of advantage taking.

At this point, the logic of self-interest takes over, to the public good. Each side to the transaction will surrender those things that it values only if it receives in exchange things to which it attaches a greater value. Each voluntary exchange leaves both sides better off than they were before. Because there are no obvious negative externalities (who is hurt because A's children get better care?), the private gains to the parties are also translated into social gains. An extensive system of contracts, in which all contracts share this feature of mutual gain, should—and would—lead us toward an improved social state of affairs. Each individual exchange has led to an improvement of the welfare of the parties to the exchange. As that process is repeated many times, the impact of the improvements is cumulative. At the end of the process, each person should be better off than he or she was at the outset, with nobody being left worse off. Because everyone is better off in the final state of the world than in the original one, there is a social optimum, which can even be measured by the exacting standards of Pareto optimality.[5]

In practice, matters will not be perfect, of course, because contracts are costly to negotiate, to draft, and to enforce.[6] There comes a point at which the transaction costs of making new bargains exceed the gains that anyone could hope to derive from them. The system will therefore reach equilibrium before all potential gains from trade are exhausted. Transaction costs will prevent some worthwhile exchanges from occurring. Nevertheless, this limitation on social welfare is a fact of life that can be overcome only by devising cheaper modes of contracting (for example, group contracts), which allow more bargains to go forward. It is hardly a reason for striking down those contracts that have been able to emerge in the face of these transactional obstacles.

The Limitations on Contract

Imperfect Information

The critical issue is this: Is there any reason why this system of bargaining is inappropriate for medical malpractice cases, both generally and in the special case of obstetrics and gynecology? Several reasons can be offered. It could be argued that individuals do not have sufficient information to decide which bargains are in their best interests. There is surely reason for concern here, but the problem may be overstated. Initially, the difficulties operate in both directions. If individuals have imperfect information, then so do regulators, administrators, juries, and judges. To treat the question as though imperfect information runs only in one direction is to misstate the universal problems with imperfect information. Both forms of imperfect information—that of the consumer and that of the regulator—are critical. Furthermore, where public regulation is involved, a single set of rules must work for all those affected, notwithstanding any individual differences in taste and demand. The rules, moreover, will be prepared by persons who have no real information about the subjective preferences of the people whom they wish to protect.

Looking then to consumers, we can assume that they make decisions with imperfect information. That is not the same, however, as their having no information at all. Moreover, in the case of consumers the incentive structures are more favorable than for others involved because the individuals who seek to get information are obtaining it for themselves, not for the public at large. People can make inquiries, rely on systems of public certification, do business with institutions that have substantial reputations, and hire intermediates to make certain decisions about who shall provide what kind of health care. The rise of health maintenance organizations (HMOs), group insurance, employer and union plans, and medical advertising represents increased efforts to close the information gap at a reasonable cost.[7] Surely, no one believes that the problems of information are so great that patients should be denied the right to choose their own physicians because patients do not have medical degrees (or because they do!). Furthermore, no one believes that the right is valueless because the choice is at best random.

In general, imperfect information is a cost. Just as with other costs, market institutions that are designed to reduce those costs will arise to the extent that these institutions are cost justified. Typically, individual patients will decide to trade off some measure of independence and some resources to get some but not all of the information they need. Even today, patients use the patchwork system to select hospitals and physicians, if only because it is better than any alternative that can be devised. It is far from obvious, therefore, that a contract system must founder badly in choosing the rules to govern malpractice. Why allow freedom in the selection of physicians but not in the choice of malpractice rules?

Medical mishaps are a common occurrence, and the issue has been widely addressed in the press. People therefore contract with the expectation of gain but with the knowledge of possible loss, especially in the medical setting. A set of rules for allocating the loss of that failure is not currently negotiated because there is no freedom of contract in that domain. Let that freedom be guaranteed, and the subject will not be some idle afterthought to the basic negotiations. Very serious attention will be given to the types of terms that can and should be imposed with respect to the potential loss. Any institution must have terms favorable enough to attract patients, yet the terms cannot be so one-sided as to bankrupt those patients at the back end if and when something goes wrong. Whenever contracts are used, both sides have to trade off gain against loss, benefit against inconvenience. For large institutions, the fact that some level of medical malpractice will occur should be accepted as a social given. There are too many cases for all to be handled correctly, no matter what level of care is taken. The task of contracting is not only to reduce these bad cases but also to see that the handling of bad cases does not overwhelm the system as a whole.

Today, there is extensive competition for the provision of medical services. That competition need not be confined to matters of price, thereby holding the minimum level of acceptable services constant by government edict. There can also be competition over the level of compensation that will be provided in the event of a medical mishap. Terms that regulate liability for medical mishaps do not have to be kept apart from the general market processes by which agreements for medical and hospital services are formed. Experimentation and innovation are possible here. The critic who thinks that an adoption of contractual freedom automatically means that medical providers will exclude all liability for all untoward consequences should ask himself how he would respond when a rival provider offers some package of benefits to persons injured during the course of medical treatment. Surely, such a medical provider would not remain idle as market share and profits shrink.

In the abstract it is hard to determine the precise set of optimal terms for all medical situations. Nevertheless, it is fairly clear that the present set of legal rules is not optimal, given the decision of many professionals to leave the market,[8] the incentives for excessive care that liability rules can create, and the enormous litigation costs of the system at large. The fine tuning that is needed to improve the rules cannot be done by juries and courts who are years behind the times and who totally lack the hands-on experience necessary to make the relevant trade-offs. Contract solutions, on the other hand, lead to decentralization and to the quicker dissemination of successful practices and business arrangements throughout the medical profession.

Binding the Child

There is one important qualification that applies to obstetrical (but not gynecological) care: the physician-patient relationship is between the physician and the woman, yet the losses may be suffered by a third party, the unborn child, who may be condemned by poor medical treatment to lead a life of diminished capacity and chronic pain. The presence of this third party provides an obvious challenge to the contract model, with its central tenet that two parties cannot bind a stranger through their own agreement. It is plausible, therefore, that no contract between a medical provider and a woman (with or without the child's father) could bind the infant, who surely has not given any consent of his or her own.

A moment's reflection, however, should be sufficient to dispel any illusion that the prohibition against binding strangers by contract applies to the parent-child context. It is true that small children, not to say unborn children, cannot contract on their own behalf; nor have they consented to the tort rules or their no-fault substitutes. The way to escape the difficulties of consent, however, is not with an elaborate network of state decrees. Rather, the institution of guardianship solves the consent problem, primarily by ensuring that the people with the right incentives contract on behalf of the young. Parents, by virtue of their status, have obligations not to abuse or neglect an infant and, furthermore, incur affirmative obligations of support. These obligations surely begin with the labor and nourishment that parents should provide their offspring, but they are not so limited. Parents may also contract with third parties for the benefit of their children, just as they do when they buy their children food at the supermarket or provide for their education at a public or private school.

The role of guardianship is deemphasized by those who are unsympathetic to contract solutions. Atiyah writes accordingly, "Babies and children are also consumers of health care, and it is a serious question whether the law should allow the rights of children to tort standards of medical care to be bargained away on their behalf by adults."[9] The argument loses its emotive force when it is made clear that not just any "adult" has the power to so bargain. The real question is whether children are better off under the present tort regime, created by judges and legislators, than they would be under the alternative contract regime, in which their parents would determine what is in their best interests. If parents are willing to accept the same terms that are applicable to their children, then there is good reason to think that the contract rules will be superior to the tort rules now said to protect the children. It is very hard to see how parents can systematically exploit their children when they agree to the same types of legal risks that their children must face. But even in cases in which the contract terms are different (because the medical procedures are different), we should be very slow to condemn the variation as a parental sellout of the child's interest. Calling the issue of parental control a "serious question," as Atiyah does, only reaffirms that the issue is important, a point on which everyone can agree. It does not indicate, however, how the question should be resolved. The greater conflict of interest is between the child and the state, not between the child and the parent.

As a matter of sheer necessity, the guardianship arrangement dominates issues of medical care. There is little doubt, for example, that parental consent is what energizes the selection of and payment for medical services. It can also work for liability. If parents can make all other fundamental decisions about the provision of medical care, then why should one element of that set of choices—the terms of compensation if matters go awry—be immune from parental choice? Under the current medical malpractice system, parents are entitled to choose any contingent-fee lawyer to bring suits on behalf of their minor children. Why, then, should they be powerless to contract out of that tort system for the benefit of their children? After the fact, some parents may regret that choice, just as they regret other decisions made on other matters. Yet here, as elsewhere, liability rules should be fashioned with an eye not only to compensation ex post but also to ensuring the access of medical services at affordable prices ex ante. The only variation required in the traditional scheme of contracting with regard to medical liabilities to newborns is the recognition of the guardianship relation. That is hardly an innovation of modern legal theory.

To be sure, there are occasions when the state will override the preferences of parents with regard to their children. These cases, however, fall rather clearly within the traditional area of abuse or neglect. How else should we view a decision to refuse surgical treatment to remove intestinal blockage of a Down's syndrome child or (of only somewhat more difficulty) to refuse to give to a child medical treatment that is inconsistent with the religious beliefs of the parents? Again, the ordinary decisions on how to seek medical care are today most emphatically within the province of the parents, whose natural instincts provide the best shield that most children can ever hope to obtain. Likewise, parents are in the best position to address liability issues on behalf of their children.

Access for the Poor

It may be argued that these contract arguments work for the middle class but do not begin to address the question of access to medical care for indigent families and their children. The concern is that indigent persons, because of their inferior economic status, bring less bargaining power to the contractual negotiations. This point misses the source of current concern by failing to understand the intimate relationship between access to medical care and tort liability for malpractice. The use of the wrong liability terms has and will continue to have a powerful adverse effect on the level of care made available to people who cannot afford to purchase it. This point can be brought home most clearly if we consider the position of a hospital that supplies charitable care to indigent patients free of charge. Historically, these hospitals have, as part of their admissions provisions, included conditions that exempted themselves from any and all liability for physician or hospital negligence.[10] These clauses have typically been struck down as an improper form of contractual exploitation of the extraordinary bargaining strength of the hospital.[11]

Nonetheless, judicial condemnation of these charitable exemption clauses seems misconceived. With respect to indigents, public insistence that a hospital be unable to release itself from medical malpractice liability necessarily curtails access to care as a way to increase malpractice protection. Thus, let us assume that the hospital has a fixed and limited budget that it uses to alleviate the plight of the needy. In a world without any malpractice liability, the hospital could treat, for example, 1,000 patients and deliver a quality of care that results in 10 malpractice cases, for which no one receives any compensation. When the ability to contract out of liability is barred, some portion of the charitable budget must fund the potential malpractice liabilities. Let us assume, therefore, that the number of cases that can be handled decreases by 10 percent, to 900, while the incidence of malpractice decreases by more that half, to 0.433 percent. Now, there are only four such incidents.

Which world is the better world for the indigents in need of medical care? If we looked only at those persons who in fact received medical care in both instances, then the choice would seem to be clear: the patient under the malpractice regime is better off on both counts. He receives a higher standard of care, as well as some measure of compensation if this standard of care is not met. Because the patient wins both ways, the forced judicial invalidation of exculpation clauses appears fully justified.

This analysis is incomplete, however, because it ignores the position of those 100 patients who were unable to obtain care because of the restriction in access caused by the new malpractice regime. If even 10 percent of these persons suffered adverse consequences because of their inability to obtain any care, then the conclusion is reversed. The loss of access means that there are now more in the original cohort of actual and potential patients who sustain bad outcomes under the system with full tort protection than there are in the system that does not provide any protection (10 + 4 > 10). These numbers are chosen for illustrative purposes; one cannot have any confidence that the rate of failure will necessarily be greater with liability rules firmly in place. In principle, the errors could run in either direction. It is quite possible that with a medical malpractice system the amount of negligent treatment will not be cut by more than half; it may be cut by less. It is also possible that many more than 10 percent of people who are not treated will develop some serious complications. Thus, just as this scenario may be too grim, it may also be too optimistic.

It is doubtful, of course, that we shall ever obtain reliable data on the relative strength of the two effects. Nonetheless, three observations can be made about the current state of affairs. First, the concern about impaired access to medical care is a constant theme of health professionals and administrators who work with indigent patients. They report clinics closing or restricting access to service, and they cite the cost of medical malpractice insurance as one reason for the current distress. It is doubtful that they are grossly wrong in their empirical estimations.[12] Second, the leading legal decisions that deny the right of hospitals to release themselves from medical malpractice do not even address the interaction between the quality of care required and the resulting amount of care that hospitals can then provide. There is no reason, therefore, to think that they have made the correct trade-offs when they did not identify these trade-offs in the first place.[13] Third, there is little reason to think that the hospitals have any perverse institutional incentives on the liability question. The profit motive is surely not dominant in any area in which the institutional purpose is to give away services at some positive cost to itself. Charitable hospitals hardly fall into the class of fast-buck operators, fly-by-night sharpies, or gougers of the poor. It is hard to imagine that prominent donors to medical research would oppose use of their funds for medical malpractice litigation and damage costs if those expenditures produced any aggregate improvement in the overall medical care provided. There is a very large number of charitable hospitals; to the extent that these hospitals once adopted a uniform set of provisions, the set is probably based on the sensible observation that a liability regime does more harm than good to its intended beneficiaries. There is good reason to believe that they may have been right.

The advent of increased public expenditures on medical care for the poor has changed the situation. Services that were once provided for free are now (at least in principle) paid for by direct government funds. In this context poor people do not have to bargain for themselves any more than middle-class people must bargain when represented by their employers. Public officials who supply the funds can bargain on their behalf to obtain the best mix of medical access and malpractice protection. It is possible that they might want to purchase some malpractice protection for women and children, unborn and born, who are covered by their plans. These agencies face budget constraints that force them to make choices between how much money they wish to spend on preserving access and how much they wish to spend on ensuring compensation when medical care turns out to be inadequately provided. They are, of course, subject to the same bureaucratic limitations inherent in all public agencies, but if we are prepared to accept their role in other aspects of medical care, then I am hard pressed to see why they could not be allowed to contract as agents for their beneficiaries on tort liability.

Yet how would they proceed? Welfare agencies also face heavy budget constraints and must make the same trade-offs between access to the system and the level of protection afforded those lucky enough to make it into the system. The official involved might make the same decision desired by middle-class persons and therefore stipulate for some particular malpractice compensation scheme. There seems to be no reason why public agencies could not insist that all malpractice disputes go to arbitration, as can now be done by private employers.[14] Indeed, there is no reason to tie the fortunes of the poor to the tastes of the middle class. The desire for greater legal protection against medical malpractice may well reflect middle-class patients' greater willingness and ability to pay. There seems to be no reason to assume that poor people have the same preferences, given their far lower incomes; hence, poor people should not be forced to enter into exactly the same kind of contracts. I would therefore allow public officials virtually complete contractual freedom in the kinds of medical services contracts they negotiate for the poor. The argument here is not that the "no liability solution" of bygone days is necessarily best. It is that the persons in charge of the programs have better information about the optimal set of contract terms than do legislatures or courts, or even (dare one say it?) public policy analysts and law professors.

THE VIRGINIA NO-FAULT STATUTE

The Political Setting

My defense of contractual regimes for medical malpractice certainly does not represent today's dominant opinion—quite the opposite. The first question—who should decide what the rules are—is answered routinely in favor of plenary state authority. Political action focuses on the second question: what rules the state should impose. Given this particular framework, it is quite clear that the legal solutions that arise will no longer have the same type of generality, efficiency, and (if it matters) elegance of the contractual solution. The pattern of behavior will be quite different because it will now be necessary to contend with the dynamics of interest-group politics, as life-and-death questions ensure that both emotions and stakes will be high.

The first rule of politics is that general solutions are often very hard to achieve because there will be no sponsors to introduce them. Political action does not start with overarching philosophical theories. It is galvanized by crisis, by dramatic incidents, and by the sense of dire necessity. The Injured Infant Act, providing for no-fault insurance in certain obstetrical cases, is illustrative of the general process. Over the years, there have been a large number of attempts to formulate comprehensive medical no-fault proposals,[15] and these proposals have routinely foundered on the inability of anyone to define the universal class of compensable events—that is, those for which the new liabilities would be imposed—with a degree of precision that would make the system workable in the broad run of cases.[16] There have been, however, many well-publicized judgments or settlements against individual obstetricians for huge verdicts, beyond the levels of insurance they carry and perhaps beyond their net worth.[17]

Initially, there is something very wrong with a system that says to a physician: "Thank you for saving by timely and courageous intervention 99 children from terrible fates and ruined lives. You have earned your fee"; yet when the 100th child suffers one of those terrible fates (even because of negligence), we say, "Pay the full costs." The score card that summarizes the results looks odd indeed: the net benefit to society is 99 lives spared a terrible fate; the physician's routine fees in 99 cases are wiped out by the huge losses from the last case. There is a manifest divergence between the private loss that the physician bears and the net social gain that the physician's activities produce. Actions that, on balance, everyone would favor ex ante—for example, having the physician do medical procedures that succeed 99 percent of the time and negligently fail 1 percent of the time—generate financially ruinous results for the physician. The source of the gap is clear. The medical malpractice system does not explicitly credit the physician for the benefits provided in the 99 cases of successful medical intervention. Yet individuals in making private decisions of whether to accept or reject medical care will regard that benefit as *more important* than whether compensation will be forthcoming ex post for the tiny fraction of cases that go wrong.[18]

The question that emerges in the legal system is this: Once the medical malpractice system puts the wrong rules for compensation in place in the obstetrical area, what can be done to undo the damage? Private responses are surely possible, although not ideal. Fees can be raised to cover the mishaps, but they are limited by the wealth of the patients, a dominant concern for many indigent patients. Moreover, patients' wealth limits the purchase of additional safety precautions. If the situation gets bad enough, the movement will then be for legislation, which is what apparently prompted the passage of the Virginia Injured Infant Act.[19] A close look at this novel statute reveals some of the compromises that had to be made to secure its passage and some of the serious defects in its basic structure.[20]

The Statutory Design

The Virginia Injured Infant Act is restricted to one class of major injury:

"Birth-related neurological injury" means injury to the brain or spinal cord of an infant caused by the deprivation of oxygen or mechanical injury occurring in the course of labor, delivery, or resuscitation in the immediate post-delivery period in a hospital which renders the infant permanently nonambulatory, aphasic, incontinent, and in need of assistance in all phases of daily living.[21]

The statute provides measures to collect and distribute the funds necessary to handle this important class of cases. First, the disposition of claims is taken out of the tort system (with its jury trials) and placed before the State Industrial Commission,[22] whose usual responsibility is to hear workers' compensation claims, which themselves often raise substantial medical issues. Second, there is a network of substantive provisions. Most notably, funds for the program are raised by a per capita flat fee of $5,000 for individual obstetricians who choose to participate in the program.[23] This fee is fixed by statute for the first year[24] and cannot be raised in subsequent years, apparently even for inflation.[25] The fee for hospitals is $50 per delivery per year, subject to an overall cap of $150,000 per hospital.[26] Physicians who do not participate in this program are nonetheless required to contribute $250 per year to the fund.[27] If the funds raised from these three sources are insufficient to cover the obligations of the program, the resultant shortfall will be covered by taxes levied on all insurance companies within the state, whether or not they are in the business of providing coverage for medical malpractice.[28]

As to the distribution of benefits from the plan, the patterns of compensation that have been adopted parallel those used in workers' compensation plans. The statute provides no compensation for pain and suffering;[29] it provides limited compensation for lost earnings, based on 50 percent of the average weekly wage, as well as compensation for medical and other support services over the life of the program, with setoffs, dollar for dollar, for collateral sources under the plan.[30]

Participation in the program is not mandatory for physicians or hospitals. They are permitted to opt into the system at will. If they agree to participate, however, the quality of services they provide is subject to review by a board of directors, which administers the Injured Infant Act.[31] The physicians and hospitals must also agree to participate in developing a program to provide obstetrical care to indigent patients.[32] Curiously, neither physicians nor hospitals seem to be required to disclose to their patients their decision regarding participation in the plan.

It is instructive to compare the political solution reached by the Injured Infant Act with the solution that might be reached under market arrangements. The analysis is conveniently divided into two parts: coverage and funding.

Coverage

The coverage provisions here are restricted to only one class of serious injuries. Why is only this class included when other types of injuries might well be as serious? From the point of view of an outsider, one possible answer is that the problems arising in this class of cases were so pressing that the legislature was forced to take it specifically in hand, leaving the others to the malpractice system. Indeed, if there are an estimated 40 such cases per year,[33] the sums involved are in fact quite large. Each case under the program could easily generate present liabilities of several million dollars. Another explanation, with perhaps more descriptive power, is that the compromise was necessary to get the bill through the Virginia legislature. Trial lawyers form a powerful interest group in all states, and they could well have blocked the more general removal of all obstetrical cases from the medical malpractice system (after all, they do not want a precedent that ends malpractice suits altogether).

A contract solution would doubtless be more general in its coverage. Ex ante, the dominant question is whether both sides are better off by taking cases out of the tort system and providing some alternative system for compensation. Costs of prevention, needs for compensation ex post, and administrative costs of the system are likely to control that inquiry. If that is the case, then there seems to be little reason to differentiate by source within the class of severe injuries. Although it may not be clear exactly how all severe injuries would be covered, it is a good guess that they would all be covered in the same way.

There is also a question as to whether this choice of compensable events to be covered by the statute makes sense. Here, the definition on its face appears quite narrow, being restricted to "injury to the brain or spinal cord of an infant caused by the deprivation of oxygen or mechanical injury occurring in the course of labor, deliver, or resuscitation."[34] The operative concern is not semantic because the meaning of the terms is as clear as good legal draftsmanship can make it. Instead, the issue is an empirical one: What is the percentage of all birth defect cases that will be contestable under the definition? To answer this question, one must know a great deal more about medicine than any outsider to the profession knows. Nonetheless, it is possible to at least note two sources of concern that might be raised about this warranty.[35]

First, it is often difficult to distinguish serious injuries caused at or before birth from those caused by birth defects. The ultimate physical condition that results is often the same in either case (for example, brain damage), although the medical evidence is not reliable enough for anyone to make an accurate determination of causation. Second, it may be that certain serious fetal injuries can be caused by intermittent drug (for example, cocaine) use, which could not be distinguished from the compensable injuries covered under the statute. Here, the problem turns out to be especially acute because there now seem to be ample data suggesting that even a single "hit" of cocaine in the first trimester of pregnancy can cause massive neurological damage, even though it might be very difficult to trace the results thereafter.[36] Moreover, the incidence of maternal use of illegal drugs, including cocaine, during early pregnancy is very high: it is estimated to be as much as 11 percent.[37] Under a system of negligence liability, it is unlikely that even a tiny fraction of these cases would create a colorable case for liability. Under the Virginia statute, however, all of them do, especially if there is no trace of cocaine or any other illegal drug left in the child's system six months later when birth occurs. It seems most unlikely that the Virginia no-fault plan was intended to be a compensation program for victims of maternal drug abuse—yet that is the risk it creates.

The Injured Infant Act seeks to handle these problems by using rebuttable presumptions: "A rebuttable presumption shall arise that the injury alleged is a birth-related neurological injury where it has been demonstrated, to the satisfaction of the Industrial Commission, that the infant has sustained a brain or spinal cord injury caused by oxygen deprivation or mechanical injury."[38] The initial presumption appears to be set in favor of the physician until the commission makes the critical finding (which should not be made in drug cases) that the brain or spinal cord injury is attributable to oxygen deprivation or spinal injury. Yet that question of fact can be highly controverted, and although presumptions can shift burdens, they do little to reduce total error. At most, presumptions only determine whether the large residual errors that uncertainty creates are borne mainly by plaintiffs or defendants. The drug cases could still arise with sufficient frequency to inundate the entire system. If the gray area under the statute turns out to be very large for medical reasons, then clarity of draftsmanship will offer no refuge from an administrative nightmare or from the strategic maneuvers of both sides.

Other complications may also arise. Thus, the claimant who thinks negligence is clear will try to keep the case outside the statute, whereas the defendant will try to bring it within the statute. Yet nothing in the statute deals with this reversal of roles, which is familiar to lawyers who work in workers' compensation cases. Ironically, a negligence standard, for all its flaws, may turn out to be more desirable, if only because fewer cases straddle the negligence-no negligence line than straddle the iatrogenic injury-birth defect or drug usage line. Under the statute, we have no market information and hence no capacity for incremental adjustments in the basic rules. There will have to be another obstetrical crisis before corrective action can be taken.

Funding

Equally striking are the provisions of the statute that address the funding of the system as a whole. In market settings any contract must work for the joint benefit of the parties. There may be an uneven distribution of the gains from trade, but each side will garner at least some portion of those gains. Ex ante, there should be no losers. Legislation must not satisfy that constraint, especially as the constitutional safeguards to economic liberties and property today are set at a very low level indeed.[39] Hence, we should expect to see large amounts of wealth redistribution take place within the system.

Initially, the fees charged do not begin to approximate the risks covered. The Injured Infant Act does not reveal a budget estimate as to the total likely expenses, which is then made the target for the total charges imposed on the participants in the system. Quite the opposite: the statute contemplates that any shortfall that may develop shall be covered by all insurance carriers within the state, regardless of the lines of business they write. Here, the physicians as a group are able to impose huge contingent (but very real) liabilities on insurance carriers who write only other, unrelated lines of business. The provision that insulates plan participants from any historically justified rate increases makes it clear that the real question is not whether but when the contingent liability will kick in. This financing decision is not without its negative allocative consequences. The imposition of taxes always distorts market decisions in the goods or commodities that are taxed. When unrelated lines of insurance are subject to taxes, they become less available to the consumers who benefit from them because the tax drives from the marketplace all transactions in which the difference between the buyer's gain and the seller's cost is less than the tax in question.[40] Large taxes therefore tend to produce large misallocations. Insurance companies are an easy populist target for attack, and their customers are too diffuse to protest. The statutory financing scheme therefore exports misery—it does not eliminate it.

The usual somber conclusion of the public choice literature holds here.[41] Efforts in the political process to correct one distortion, such as the medical malpractice tort rules, only create other distortions in other markets. The wisest sage cannot hazard a guess as to which set of distortions is greater. The ordinary analyst can say with confidence that competitive markets in both sectors yield a better social solution.

The redistribution provided by the statute works in more than one direction. To extract profits from insurance companies, the obstetrician groups had to make deals with other legislative interest groups, and they did. With which groups the deal was made is hard for an outsider to determine. But surely welfare and children's rights groups and some segments of the medical and insurance industries are likely candidates. The evidence appears on the face of the statute. The definition of a participating physician or hospital includes only those willing to participate in developing programs to assist the poor: limited public service has become the quid pro quo for reduced tort liability. I do not wish to quarrel with public assistance as such. But why should it be funded from special taxes on obstetricians and hospitals?

In a sense the odd funding of this statute is a quid pro quo for getting out of the tort system, which obstetricians and hospitals never should have entered. The new principle is that bad common law rules are corrected only if the losers pay tribute to the legislature that relieves them of their pains. (It is as if justice is done when the thief agrees to sell back stolen property to its owner at a below-market price.) The Byzantine system of indirect payments that emerges results only in public mischief because no one must ever make an explicit public reckoning of what resources should go to welfare generally, or why. The political system thus generates a set of hidden taxes and off-budget appropriations with which no citizen can keep pace.[42] How ironic it is that private contracts are attacked on the ground that consumers have imperfect information! The Virginia statute is drafted in a way to keep its real costs hidden from public view.

Not only does the redistribution worked by the statute take place between sectors but it also occurs within the medical sector. Physicians are forced to contribute to the plan, whether or not they benefit from participation; yet in ordinary private insurance markets, there are powerful incentives to differentiate costs of coverage for different insureds.[43] The insurance company that can identify low-risk providers of medical services and offer them premiums to match those services will eliminate any implicit subsidy of inefficient producers by efficient producers. The legislated insistence on a flat fee prevents this particular program from having its desired effect. Now, physicians with routine practices are forced to subsidize their colleagues who specialize in high-risk pregnancies. Moreover, the same implicit redistribution can take place, for example, between small community hospitals that do not derive any benefit from the hospital cap and large university hospitals, with a far riskier patient mix, that do. In principle these subsidies are all inefficient, and, at least with respect to institutions, the plan should be modified to allow experience rating if the data proves reliable enough to sustain it.

What about the consumer of medical services? In one sense, the statute in question does not mark a move to consumer consent. The physician or hospital can opt into this system at will, but it appears that the statute does not even require them to inform their patients of the choice. At the very least, a provision that requires clear disclosure would be some improvement, because medical providers would have to gauge the effect of their choices on their ability to maintain their practices. Even if the patients should unanimously approve the abandonment of the malpractice system, however, one could not be confident that the system represents a social improvement, given the huge implicit subsidies (especially from insurers and less so from nonparticipating physicians) built into the plan.

CONCLUSION

It is not clear whether in the aggregate this no-fault situation is better or worse than the malpractice situation it replaced. That malpractice system tended to make every serious birth injury a tort suit, so that the skilled specialist physicians and large hospitals suffered disproportionate losses. This no-fault system hopes to correct that set of distortions, but in the process creates another, equally serious, if not more serious, set of distortions. The point here is not that the no-fault system is not perfect; no system is. Rather, it is that the system, especially with active legislative intervention, is more politically charged, and more imperfect, than it need be.

Relative to Virginia's Injured Infant Act, markets have two great strengths that are often underappreciated. First, they allow some experimentation for ideal contractual terms, which could provide for solutions better than those of either the medical malpractice system or its limited no-fault alternative. Second, markets weed out all the implicit subsidies that legislatures and interest groups are routinely able to work into their deals. These advantages are not simply abstract or theoretical. They increase the capacity of the society to provide needed goods and services for all its citizens. In the clamor for short-term reform, the overall social effects are often ignored in favor of more insistent, and more parochial, considerations. Two wrongs do not make a right. State-mandated no-fault statutes are not the right response to the blunders of the present malpractice system. Markets are.

REFERENCES AND NOTES

1. This was the year of the first major physician revolt against malpractice insurance premium increases in such major states as California, Illinois, and New York. See Kotulak, R. 1975. Malpractice suits—Growing sickness. Chicago Tribune. May 11, p. 1; Malpractice: MD's revolt. 1975. Newsweek. June 9, p. 59.
2. See Havighurst, C. 1975. Medical adversity insurance: Has its time come? Duke Law J. 75:1233; Havighurst, C., and L. Tancredi. 1974. Medical adversity insurance: A no-fault approach to medical malpractice and quality assurance. Insur. Law J. 613:69.
3. Va. Code Ann. §§ 38.2-5000 to 38.2-5021 (Supp. 1987).
4. I have defended this system more fully in Epstein, R. 1977. Contracting out of the medical malpractice crisis. Perspect. Biol. Med. 20:228; Epstein, R. 1978. Medical malpractice: Its cause and cure. In The Economics of Medical Malpractice, S. Rottenberg, ed. Washington, D.C.: American Enterprise Institute, p. 245; Epstein, R. 1976. Medical malpractice: The case for contract. Am. Bar Found. Res. J. 76:87. For other defenses of the same position, see Danzon, P. M. 1985. Medical Malpractice: Theory, Evidence, and Public Policy. Cambridge, Mass.: Harvard University Press; Robinson, G. 1986. Rethinking the allocation of medical malpractice risks between patients and providers. Law Contemp. Prob. 49:173.
5. For a discussion of this exacting Pareto standard, and the alternative Kaldor-Hicks standard, whereby there is a social improvement if the winners *in principle* can compensate the losers for their pains out of their winnings from the transaction, see Coleman, J. L. 1980. Efficiency, utility, and wealth maximization. Hofstra Law Rev. 8:509. Note that the system of contracting, with its unanimous consent, satisfies both criteria and does not require any very subtle social analysis to determine the relative impacts of complex regulatory programs on both winners and losers.
6. For a formal introduction of transaction costs into modern legal and economic thinking, see, generally, Coase, R. 1960. The problem of social cost. J. Law Econ. 3:1.
7. See Danzon. 1985, p. 211; see note 4.
8. See Lewis-Idema, D. In this volume.
9. Atiyah, P. S. 1986. Medical malpractice and the contract/tort boundary. Law Contemp. Prob. 49:287, 295.

10. For example, the Supreme Court of California examined the following admissions release form in *Tunkl* v. *Regents of the University of California,* 60 Cal. 2d 92, 383 P.2d 441, 32 Cal. Rptr. 33 (1963):

> RELEASE: The hospital is a nonprofit, charitable institution. In consideration of the hospital and allied services to be rendered and the rates charged therefor, the patient or his legal representative agrees to and hereby releases The Regents of the University of California, and the hospital from any and all liability for the negligent or wrongful acts or omissions of its employees, if the hospital has used due care in selecting its employees.

> Ibid. at 94, 383 P.2d at 442, 32 Cal. Rptr. at 34.

11. Thus, the California court struck down the clause in *Tunkl* (see note 10). In his opinion for the court, Justice Tobriner reasoned:

> Thus the attempted but invalid exemption involves a transaction which exhibits some or all of the following characteristics. It concerns a business of a type generally thought suitable for public regulation. The party seeking exculpation is engaged in performing a service of great importance to the public, which is often a matter of practical necessity for some members of the public. The party holds himself out as willing to perform this service for any member of the public who seeks it, or at least for any member coming within certain established standards. As a result of the essential nature of the service, in the economic setting of the transaction, the party invoking exculpation possesses a decisive advantage of bargaining strength against any member of the public who seeks his services. In exercising a superior bargaining power the party confronts the public with a standardized adhesion contract of exculpation, and makes no provision whereby a purchaser may pay additional reasonable fees and obtain protection against negligence. Finally, as a result of the transaction, the person or property of the purchaser is placed under the control of the seller, subject to the risk of carelessness by the seller or his agents.

> Ibid. at 98–101, 383 P.2d at 445–446, 32 Cal. Rptr. at 37–38.

12. This was a constant theme in the discussion sessions at the symposium. Few of the speakers who made this assertion had a strong intellectual orientation toward markets.

13. See *Madden* v. *Kaiser Foundation Hospitals,* 17 Cal. 3d 699, 552 P.2d 1178, 131 Cal. Rptr. 882 (1976). Note that insurance companies are often unwilling to provide additional coverage against loss for an additional premium because of the risk of adverse selection—that is, those persons who are likely to demand the coverage are the most likely to sue. The practice, therefore, is to make the coverage constant across broad classes of cases. See Epstein, R., C. Gregory, and H. Kalven, Jr., eds. 1987 Supp. Cases and Materials on Torts. Boston: Little, Brown, p. 44, note 3.

14. Carter Phillips, speaking on behalf of the American Medical Association (joined by 32 other medical groups), made this point very clear in his oral presentation at the symposium (see his and Elizabeth Esty's chapter, this volume). Phillips, like me, is doubtful that any major restructuring of medical malpractice laws can be limited solely to obstetrics and gynecology.

15. See, for example, the sources cited in note 2.

16. See, for example, Abraham, K. S. 1987. Individual action and collective responsibility: The dilemma of mass tort reform. Va. Law Rev. 73:845, 886–889; Keeton, R. E. 1973. Compensation for medical accidents. Univ. Pa. Law Rev. 121:590, 605, 612–614.

17. For example, a $10 million verdict against three prominent obstetricians in Washington, D.C., prompted their patients and colleagues to rally around them on appeal. The verdict exhausted the obstetricians' insurance coverage and, if it had been upheld on

appeal, may have forced them into bankruptcy (Lee Hockstader, Colleagues rally for 3 doctors ordered to pay $10 million. 1988. Washington Post. June 4, p. A-1). The case, however, was settled for $4 million—the limit of the obstetricians' coverage—as well as for $800,000 paid separately by the hospital (Lee Hockstader. King of area malpractice cases creates stir in, out of court. 1988. Washington Post. September 10, p. B-1).

18. Clearly, this numerical example is dependent on the assumption that most medical interventions today are beneficial. That assumption seems to be unquestionable, even if the exact ratio is subject to doubt. But even if the number were 98 to 2, the net positive would still be very large, and the analytical point would remain the same. Benefits conferred are not ignored in any ex ante calculation. In addition, if the percentage of negligence cases were much higher, then the system would collapse under its weight. The frequency of malpractice litigation would be unbearable if, for example, 2 percent of surgeries resulted in malpractice litigation. If the average surgeon performed 100 surgeries per year, there would be two cases per year. If each suit lasted five years, the average surgeon would be a defendant in 10 cases at one time. Even the present frequency of litigation is far lower than this.

It has been suggested that the real torts crisis is that too few victims sue. See Abel, R. L. 1987. The real tort crisis—Too few claims. Ohio State Law J. 48:443–467. Abel relies on the work of Patricia Danzon, showing that 90 percent of the incidents of medical negligence do not result in any legal action (ibid., p. 448, citing Danzon. 1985, pp. 19–21, 23; see note 4). Danzon's figures suggest that in 1974 there was a nationwide total of 260,000 negligently inflicted injuries out of more than 1.5 million iatrogenic injuries (Danzon. 1985, p. 20). If all these injuries resulted in suits, as Abel urges, it would overwhelm the system.

19. For a commentary on this article that reveals the ideas and pressures underlying the initial drafting of the Injured Infant Act, see O'Connell, J. 1988. Pragmatic constraints on market approaches: A response to Professor Epstein. Va. Law Rev. 74:1475.

20. For a fuller discussion of the content and passage of the statute, see Note, innovative no-fault tort reform for an endangered specialty. 1988. Va. Law Rev. 74:1487.

21. Va. Code Ann. § 38.2-5001 (Supp. 1987) [hereafter referred to by section number only].

22. § 38.2-5003.

23. § 38.2-5019(A)(1).

24. Ibid.

25. § 38.2-5020(A).

26. § 38.2-5019(A)(2).

27. §§ 38.2-5019(A)(3) to 38.2-5020(A).

28. § 38.2-5020(B). The collections are made "if required to maintain the Fund on an actuarially sound basis."

29. § 38.2-5009.

30. Ibid.

31. § 38.2-5001. "As appointed by the Governor of Virginia, the Board shall consist of a general citizen's representative and of representatives of the other interest groups under the plan— participating hospitals, participating physicians, liability insurers, and nonparticipating physicians—such that the majority of the Board represents its participants" (§ 38.2- 5016).

32. § 38.2-5001. It is certainly worth noting that the obligation to participate in such an effort is not made a separate substantive provision of the statute but is incorporated into the definition of a "participating" physician or hospital.

33. See Heland, K. V. 1987. Memorandum to the American College of Obstetricians and Gynecologists, Committee on Professional Responsibility. March 5 (on file with the Virginia Law Review Association).

34. § 38.2-5001.

35. These issues were raised in a discussion at the symposium by Donald N. Medearis, Jr., Charles Wilder Professor of Pediatrics at Harvard Medical School and chief of the Children's Service at Massachusetts General Hospital, and Ruth Watson Lubic, general director of the Maternity Center Association, New York City.

36. According to one commentator:

> In fact, the research suggests that a single cocaine "hit" during pregnancy can cause lasting fetal damage. While a single dose of cocaine and its metabolites clear out of an adult body within 48 hours, an unborn baby is exposed for four or five days. . .
>
> Cocaine, which is soluble in fat, readily crosses the placenta, where the baby's body converts a significant portion of it to norcocaine, a water-soluble substance that does not leave the womb and that is even more potent than cocaine. Norcocaine is excreted into the amniotic fluid, which the fetus swallows, re- exposing itself to the drug. As a result, the researchers believe, almost no cocaine-exposed baby fully escapes its damaging effects.

> Brody, J. E. 1988. Cocaine: Litany of fetal risks grows. New York Times (Chicago ed.). September 6, p. 19.

37. Ibid., pp. 19, 23.

38. § 38.2-5008(1).

39. For the modern statement, see *Usery* v. *Turner Elkhorn Mining Co.*, 428 U.S. 1 (1975). I have criticized this approach at length in Epstein, R. 1985. Takings: Private Property and the Power of Eminent Domain. Cambridge, Mass.: Harvard University Press, pp. 256–258, and more briefly in Epstein, R. 1986. Self-interest and the Constitution. J. Legal Educ. 37:153, and Epstein, R. 1984. Judicial activism: Reckoning of two types of error. Cato J. 4:711.

40. For a discussion of the so-called excess burden of taxation, see Gwartney, J., and R. Stroup. 1987. Economics: Private and Public Choice, 4th ed. San Diego: Harcourt Brace Jovanovich, pp. 110–111.

41. For the classical elaboration, see Buchanan, J., and G. Tullock. 1962. The Calculus of Consent: Logical Foundations of Constitutional Democracy. Ann Arbor: University of Michigan Press. For the modern controversy, see Symposium on the theory of public choice. 1988. Va. Law Rev. 74:167–177.

42. For a related discussion concerning AIDS, see Epstein, R. 1988. The AIDS Commission's hidden tax. Wall Street Journal. June 13, p. 12.

43. For a general account of the operation of private insurance markets with respect to liability, see Epstein, R. 1985. Products liability as an insurance market. J. Legal Stud. 14:645–669; Schwartz, S. 1988. Proposals for product liability reform: A theoretical synthesis. Yale Law J. 97:353.

A Fault-Based Administrative Alternative for Resolving Medical Malpractice Claims: The AMA-Specialty Society Medical Liability Project's Proposal and Its Relevance to the Crisis in Obstetrics

CARTER G. PHILLIPS, J.D.,
AND ELIZABETH H. ESTY, J.D.*

To appreciate the nature and scope of the crisis in medical malpractice in recent years, it is necessary to consult a variety of sources that highlight different elements of the crisis. Some research has demonstrated the staggering costs of liability insurance to physicians: $60 million in 1960, compared with nearly $5 billion in 1985.[1] Other research has focused on the magnitude of malpractice awards: from 1985 through 1987, the average malpractice verdict in the Miami area was nearly $900,000, compared with the $264,000 average award in all tort cases in that area.[2] Still other research has looked at the escalating number of claims: up from 1.3 claims per 100 doctors in 1960 to more than 15 per 100 by 1987.[3]

Startling as these numbers are, it is the impact of the crisis on the public's access to medical care that changes it from a physicians' problem to a social problem. Access problems occur most frequently in the field of obstetrics. As documented by other commentators in this volume, physicians have been forced by the medical liability crisis to withdraw from the practice of obstetrics. For example, 44 percent of the counties in Georgia,[4] 42 percent of the counties in Alabama,[5] and 30 percent of the counties in Colorado[6] no longer have any physician—

---

* The authors were consultants to the AMA-Specialty Society Medical Liability Project in designing the administrative system discussed in this article. The views expressed by the authors do not necessarily reflect the views of the project itself.

either an obstetrician or family practitioner—providing obstetrical services because of the prohibitively high cost of malpractice insurance.

The most recent membership survey conducted by the American College of Obstetricians and Gynecologists (ACOG) documents the widespread impact of the current malpractice climate on the provision of obstetrical care. According to the survey, obstetrician-gynecologists (ob-gyns) increasingly are turning away from the practice of obstetrics or are limiting the portion of their practice that is devoted to high-risk obstetrical patients.[7]

The survey found that almost one in eight ob-gyns has stopped delivering babies because of concern over malpractice suits, with two-thirds of that group quitting obstetrics before the age of 55. The survey also found that 27 percent of ob-gyns now limit their care of women with high-risk pregnancies, a percentage that has increased from 23 percent in 1985 and 18 percent in 1983. Even more dramatic, in 1987, 45.4 percent of ob-gyns—up from 1.6 percent in 1985—reported that they devote 10 percent or less of their practice to high-risk care. The decreased access to obstetrical care is compounded by the fact that those who continue to practice obstetrics must devote an increasing amount of time to responding to malpractice claims: in 55 percent of all cases reported in the survey, it took three or more years to close the claim.

THE NEED FOR DRAMATIC CHANGE

The drastic situation in the field of obstetrics today illustrates how the tort reforms of the late 1970s have failed to remedy defects in the civil justice system for resolving medical liability disputes. Efforts to make changes in the traditional system—for example, allowing offsets to awards for amounts received from collateral sources and employing pretrial screening panels—have done little to alleviate the cycle of uncertainty and escalating awards that has driven the cost of malpractice insurance out of the reach of physicians in some geographic areas and in some specialties and has increased the cost of medical care for patients.[8] The failings of the current tort system have also become increasingly apparent to a wide array of groups, including the Twentieth Century Fund,[9] the AFL-CIO,[10] the American Bar Association,[11] the New York Governor's Advisory Commission on Liability Insurance,[12] the U.S. General Accounting Office,[13] the U.S. Tort Policy Working Group,[14] and the U.S. Department of Health and Human Services.[15]

The resurgence of a crisis in medical liability in the 1980s, despite the reform efforts of the 1970s, coupled with the general scholarly view that the current tort system is seriously flawed,[16] has led some states to explore more dramatic departures from the traditional system. For example, both Virginia and Florida have recently enacted legislation establishing a no-fault compensation fund for a limited category of infants who suffer from birth-related neurological injuries.[17] Commentators have called for more extensive experiments with various alternatives to the present system, including no-fault compensation for medical injuries[18] and contractual approaches.[19] It is in response to those calls, and in recognition of the reasons that have led to them, that the American Medical Association, 31 national medical specialty societies, and the Council of Medical Specialty Societies joined together to form the AMA-Specialty Society Medical Liability Project. Table 1 lists the members of the Project, and Figure 1 shows the structure of the adjudication process.

After two years of study, the Liability Project concluded that profound changes in the mechanisms used to resolve claims of medical injury and to monitor the quality of medical care should be given serious consideration by one or more states. In particular the Project saw six major defects in the present system. First, because the legal costs of pursuing a malpractice claim are so high, the current civil trial system precludes many patients from recovery for injuries caused by medical negligence.[20] Second, the present system leads to inconsistent judgments between similarly situated patients.[21] Third, there is mounting concern that juries—one-time decision makers without any experience or training in evaluating complex medical testimony—are not well suited to the task of resolving medical liability disputes.[22] Fourth, the rapid increase in the size of malpractice awards relative to other tort awards is threatening the availability and affordability of insurance and health care, a particular problem for poor patients and those in rural areas.[23] Fifth, the civil justice system is a very inefficient way to resolve medical liability disputes, with less than half of total insurance premium dollars spent by health care providers being paid to the injured patient[24] and only half of those dollars received by the patient actually compensating him or her for injuries incurred. Finally, the Project is concerned that direct efforts to detect and eradicate substandard medical practice, which may result in malpractice, are hampered by the inadequate staffing and funding of current licensing and disciplinary boards.[26]

After reviewing the pros and cons of the full range of alternative tort reform proposals, the Project concluded that a state administrative agency, applying a negligence standard and monitoring physician practices, would be best able to respond to the deficiencies in the current system while simultaneously preserving the twin goals of tort law: compensation and deterrence. The Project believes that an administrative fault-based system has several distinct advantages over the other alternatives that have been proposed. No-fault systems, such as those proposed by Jeffrey O'Connell,[27] offend our sense of justice and individ-

TABLE 1   AMA-Specialty Society Medical Liability Project Members

American Academy of Dermatology
American Academy of Facial Plastic and Reconstructive Surgery
American Academy of Family Physicians
American Academy of Neurology
American Academy of Ophthalmology
American Academy of Orthopaedic Surgeons
American Academy of Otolaryngology-Head and Neck Surgery
American Academy of Pediatrics
American Association for Thoracic Surgery
American Association of Neurological Surgeons
American Association of Plastic Surgeons
American College of Cardiology
American College of Emergency Physicians
American College of Gastroenterology
American College of Obstetricians and Gynecologists
American College of Physicians
American College of Radiology
American College of Surgeons
American Medical Association
American Psychiatric Association
American Society of Anesthesiologists
American Society of Clinical Pathologists
American Society of Cytology
American Society of Internal Medicine
American Society of Plastic and Reconstructive Surgeons
American Urological Association
College of American Pathologists
Congress of Neurological Surgeons
Council of Medical Specialty Societies
International Society for Cardiovascular Surgery
Society for Vascular Surgery
Society of Nuclear Medicine
Society of Thoracic Surgeons

ual accountability by imposing liability on health care providers who in many instances have done everything humanly possible to treat a patient and have provided competent care but with less than perfect results. Although a no-fault system removes some of the stigma from the imposition of liability, it seems likely that health care providers and patients would continue to consider the imposition of liability as reflecting adversely on the provider's competence.

Moreover, no-fault proposals do nothing to address one of the two major goals of all tort law, namely, deterrence. Thus, the Liability Project did not pursue a no-fault plan, including the "designated compensable events" scheme,[28] because of concern that either the costs of such a system would be excessive[29] or that it would be necessary to apply strictly scheduled benefits (much like the Social Security disability

Claims Resolution Function

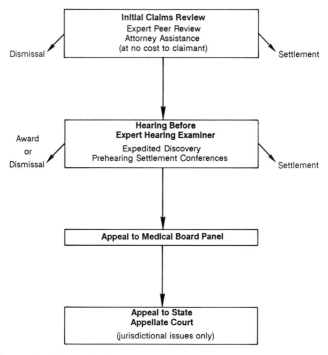

FIGURE 1.   AMA-Specialty Society Medical Liability Project Administrative Dispute Resolution System

system or the New Zealand no-fault tort system[30]) and that such guaranteed but limited benefits would be widely perceived as inadequate compensation.[31] This is not to say that the Project is opposed to the development of such alternatives; rather, it believes a fault-based administrative system could be more readily defended on the basis of available knowledge.

The private contract alternatives, such as the one discussed in this volume by Richard Epstein, were also rejected but for different reasons. First, contract proposals are predicated on an assumption that patients and health care providers are in equal bargaining positions, an assumption that is subject to serious question, particularly for most patients who have little economic bargaining power.[32]

Second, the contract proposal does nothing to ensure that medical malpractice claims are removed from the expensive and inefficient court system. Any patient who believes that he or she was injured by medical negligence and is unhappy with the bargain he or she has made ex ante is free—and likely—to enlist the assistance of a court to get the contract nullified. The very fact that the court can examine the terms of the contract to determine how it applies and whether it should be voided adds an element of uncertainty that the contract proposals were designed to eliminate.[33]

Third, it is unclear how the patient and health care provider can draft an adequate contract ex ante that will cover all situations that might develop during treatment. Although it is likely that standard contracts will be developed over time, there will always be cases with unusual or unanticipated complications. To the extent that a situation does not appear to have been contemplated under the terms of the contract, a court is likely to be persuaded to examine the terms and either find that the contract does not govern or else nullify the agreement.[34]

Finally, neither the no-fault nor the contract proposal addresses the need to improve the physician disciplinary system. Contract proposals ignore the need to improve the skills of some practitioners as an integral part of any plan to ameliorate the malpractice crisis, relying instead on the market to persuade physicians that they should maintain an appropriate level of skill.[35] Although the no-fault concept could be integrated into a comprehensive agency that also has enhanced disciplinary powers, no-fault proposals to date have focused on compensation without making any provisions for improving physician skills as a way of decreasing the incidence of medical injury. Morover, a no-fault system is explicitly not designed to uncover substandard medical practices and, therefore, will not provide information about physician practices that will enhance the disciplinary function as effectively as a fault-based system.

Nor is it reasonable to rely on any liability system alone to ensure the quality of medical care. Every study that has been done on the incidence of medical negligence has concluded that there are more instances of iatrogenic injury than there are claims of medical malpractice.[36] There is also evidence that the threat of liability alone is not an effective deterrent to inadequate medical care.[37] This evidence suggests that, whatever system for determining liability and compensation is put forth, attention must be paid separately to the question of how to effectively identify, retrain, and, where necessary, discipline physicians who are providing substandard care.

For all of these reasons, the Liability Project chose to integrate its proposal for an administrative fault-based claim into a specialized medical practices agency that would have significantly strengthened disciplinary and licensing powers. The Project urges the adoption of this model state agency on an experimental basis by one or more states. To evaluate the proposed system's ability to respond to specific problems in obstetrics, however, it is first necessary to understand how the system operates.

PROPOSAL FOR A FAULT-BASED ADMINISTRATIVE SYSTEM

Medical Practices Review Board

The proposal contemplates the establishment of a state agency—the "Medical Practices Review Board"—that will adjudicate medical liability disputes, monitor the professional performance of licensed physicians in the state, investigate substandard performance, and, if necessary, discipline physicians whose practices are inadequate.

The governing board of the agency will be appointed by the state governor (from a list of nominees selected by a nominating committee composed of representatives of legal, medical, educational, and other interest groups) and approved by the legislature. The proposal recommends a seven-person full-time board, with at least two physicians but not more than three health care professionals. The other four members cannot be health care providers; presumably one or more will be consumer representatives. This seven-member board will appoint the other key personnel in the agency, including hearing examiners, attorneys, claims reviewers, and investigators.

The Claims Resolution Process

The essence of the proposal is that claims of medical malpractice will be removed from the civil justice system and placed in a specialized administrative agency for expert and efficient resolution. This change should result in swifter and fairer dispositions of claims than is currently possible. The proposed agency will evaluate claims filed by patients and offer them the option of a state-employed attorney, who, at no cost to the patient, will present the claim in a traditional adversarial hearing to an experienced hearing examiner—instead of a jury—for decision. As described at greater length below, the claimant must demonstrate the basic legal elements of malpractice: negligence, causation, and damages. Thus, unlike the currently popular designated compensable events proposal,[38] the AMA-Specialty Society proposal is fault based. The latter proposal also differs from some of the recent congressional plans by calling for a system that operates on a state rather than a federal level.[39] Although the monitoring and disciplinary functions of the system will be limited to physicians, the adjudicatory function (malpractice claims) will encompass all health care providers as defendants: physicians, nurses, other allied health care professionals, and health care institutions such as hospitals.

The claims resolution function, which replaces the traditional jury trial system, can be divided into four stages.

Prehearing

A patient who believes that he or she has suffered an injury because of inadequate health care can initiate an administrative claim by filling out a simple form describing the circumstances that provide the basis for the claim. The claims forms will be readily available and can be completed without the assistance of an attorney. Claims reviewers (similar to present-day insurance adjusters) employed by the agency will evaluate each claim, based on a review of the medical records and interviews with the patient and any relevant health care providers.

If a claim appears to have merit, it will be submitted for review to an expert peer of the health care provider whose care has been challenged. If the peer expert also concludes that the claim has apparent merit, the board will offer to the patient the services of an attorney on its staff to litigate the claim at no charge. The patient may choose to be represented by the staff attorney or by private counsel, under terms negotiated between counsel and the patient and subject only to a review for reasonableness. If at any point during the prehearing process a claim is determined to be clearly without merit, it will be dismissed by the board. The patient may pursue such a dismissed claim by retaining a private attorney to resubmit the claim with an affidavit from an expert health care provider in the relevant field attesting that, in the expert's professional opinion, the patient's injury was, to a reasonable degree of medical certainty, caused by inadequate health care.

Hearing

After a claim passes out of the initial claims review stage, it is assigned to a hearing examiner. (The hearing examiner need not be an attorney but would be a full-time employee of the agency.) He or she will hear both medical negligence claims and disciplinary charges against physicians. The hearing examiner, much like an administrative law judge in the Social Security system, supervises cases as they develop and decides any claims that do not settle prior to the scheduled adjudicatory hearing.

To encourage reasonable and timely settlements, the proposal requires both the patient and the health care provider(s) to make blind settlement offers prior to the hearing. A party would be subject to sanctions if the outcome of the case were not an improvement over a settlement offer that the party rejected earlier. The hearing examiner will also oversee expedited discovery and ensure that both parties have valid expert evidence available to support their positions.

The hearing will be akin to a trial in that evidence will be introduced and witnesses questioned. It will be conducted in a traditional adversarial fashion, with all parties represented by attorneys. The hearing examiner may question witnesses directly and, if necessary, call independent experts for assistance. Unlike a civil trial judge, the hearing examiner will be experienced in adjudicating medical negligence claims, which will be the only kind of claims heard.

The hearing examiner will be required to render a written decision explaining the basis for the result within 90 days of the hearing. In this decision the examiner will determine whether the health care provider is liable for the patient's injury and, if so, how much should be paid in damages. Through these written decisions, the board will ensure consistency among judgments, which is expected to expedite settlements of meritorious claims by providing relatively clear reference points as to the value of similar claims. Moreover, by giving reasons for the outcome, the decisions will be more acceptable to the parties involved, as well as to physicians and laypersons generally.[40]

Board Review

The hearing examiner's decision will be subject to review by the agency's governing board, which acts like an appellate court in a trial system. The board review will be conducted by a panel of three members, one and only one of whom will be a health care provider. The board must accept the facts as found by the hearing examiner if those findings are supported by substantial evidence. (This standard is the same as that currently used in judicial appeals from decisions of administrative law judges in the Social Security disability system.) On legal issues, the panel will conduct a de novo review; that is, the panel will consider those issues anew, without any deference to the hearing examiner's determination. As a general matter, the only evidence that may be submitted to the panel is evidence relating to changed conditions (including the status of the patient) since the hearing examiner's decision.

The board will issue a written decision adopting, modifying, or rejecting the recommended judgment of the hearing examiner. If the board finds that a physician failed to provide adequate health care services, that finding will automatically be reported to a central clearinghouse. (As described at greater length below, the proposal calls for the establishment of a clearinghouse within the agency to collect information on physician practices.) A similar finding concerning any other health care professional will be reported to that professional's licensing board or other designated authority.

In addition to deciding claims that a health care provider has failed to provide adequate medical care, the board also has the authority to make rules and regulations to flesh out the statutory standards.

Judicial Review

The patient or any of the health care providers may appeal the final decision of the board to the intermediate appellate court of the state. The court's review will be very limited, looking solely at whether the board acted contrary to the statute or to its own rules, or failed to follow fair procedures. The court will thus have no authority to reexamine the facts or to hear new arguments in the case. Similarly, the court will have no authority to set medical standards or to determine whether there was medical negligence in the particular circumstances of the case. If the court concludes that the board committed an error, such as failing to provide a health care provider with the opportunity to conduct adequate cross-examination of a witness, the court will remand the case to the board. The board, as appropriate, may remand the case to the hearing examiner for further proceedings. The judicial review procedures thereby ensure that all ultimate decisions about liability and damages are made by the board.

Reforms of the Legal Rules Governing Medical Liability Determinations

In addition to restructuring the procedures for resolving malpractice claims, the proposal includes a number of modifications of the substantive legal rules for determining whether there is medical liability. The most important of the proposed reforms are summarized below.

Standard of Care

The standard of care that is applied in most states is based on the custom in the local region.[41] The AMA-Specialty Society Project proposes that the Medical Practices Review Board apply a standard that focuses on whether the challenged actions fall within a range of reasonableness, to be determined by reference to the standards of a prudent and competent practitioner in the same or similar circumstances. The board will be required to consider a variety of factors in making this determination, including the expertise of the health care provider, the state of medical knowledge, the availability of health care facilities, and reasonable access to transportation and communication facilities. This new formulation recognizes that a broad spectrum of medical care is reasonable and should not result in the imposition of liability.[42] Although it rejects the traditional locality rule, which has often made it difficult for patients to pursue valid claims against negligent health care providers, the new standard does acknowledge the role that the availability or unavailability of specialized equipment and personnel can play in the determination of what is a reasonable treatment decision in a given case.

Causation

The proposal calls for a significant modification of the legal standard for proving causation in a medical injury case. Traditionally, a patient has been required to demonstrate that it is more likely than not that the physician or other health care provider's actions caused the patient's injuries.[43] Thus, recovery would be denied unless the health care provider were more than 50 percent responsible for the patient's loss. Under the causation standard proposed by the AMA-Specialty Society Project, recovery will be permitted if the provider's negligence was a "contributing factor" in causing the injury. Damages under this standard will be apportioned according to the provider's degree of fault under a pure comparative negligence standard. This means that if the patient's preexisting condition is responsible for 60 percent of the patient's posttreatment condition and the provider's negligence is 40 percent responsible, the provider is liable for 40 percent of the damage. This causation standard is fairer to patients in that it allows them to recover even if causes other than the physician's negligence are responsible for more than 50 percent of the injuries. At the same time, it is fairer to health care professionals because it recognizes the role of preexisting conditions, usually the disease or medical status itself, in contributing to the injuries.

Informed Consent

In most states the adequacy of disclosure for informed consent is determined from the perspective of the physician or other health care provider.[44] The AMA-Specialty Society proposal adopts the current minority rule, which evaluates the adequacy of disclosure from the perspective of the reasonable patient. The Project believes that the reasonable patient standard is fairer to patients, that it will facilitate greater communication between the patient and the health care provider, and that it will lead to better, shared decision making, which will in turn help reduce the incidence of medical negligence.

Damages

The Project proposes no significant changes in current rules governing the measurement of economic damages. Economic loss will be measured by the sum of lost income plus the medical and related expenses actually incurred as a result of the injury. Unlike the current jury trial system, however, the proposed system would require damages claims (and awards) to specify the separate components of the economic damages. This requirement is designed to ensure that awards accurately reflect the losses sustained by the particular individual rather than a lump sum suggested by the claimant's attorney. It is expected that the board will develop more specific guidelines through rule making for the different components of economic damages, including interest rates, work and life expectancies, and the reasonable costs of medical services.

Noneconomic damages will be capped at an amount that is tied to a percentage of the average annual wage in the state. The cap will range from about $150,000 to $700,000, depending on the life expectancy of the patient before the injury and the extent of the patient's disability. The rule of joint and several liability will be eliminated for medical negligence claims, meaning that physicians and other health care providers will be liable for damages only in proportion to their actual responsibility for the injury. In addition, an award of future damages in excess of $250,000 at present value will be paid in accordance with a periodic payment schedule. In general, damage awards will be reduced by collateral source payments. The proposed modifications of the damages rules are designed to bring greater predictability of awards, greater rationality in the calculation of noneconomic damages, and more equitable treatment of similarly situated patients. Greater consistency in damage awards is also expected to lead to early settlement of meritorious claims.[45]

Physician Monitoring and Quality Assurance

In addition to restructuring the dispute resolution process for liability claims, the AMA-Specialty Society proposal calls for the assignment of increased powers to the Medical Practices Review Board in the area of credentialing and disciplining physicians.[46] To ensure a more comprehensive review of physician practices, the proposal includes several kinds of reporting requirements. First, hospitals will be required to review periodically the performance of all physicians with staff privileges and to report to the board's clearinghouse any finding that a physician's performance has been substandard. Second, insurers will be required to report denials of coverage for reasons that are not class based. Third, physicians who are not otherwise affiliated with an institution that conducts the required credentialing review will be required to participate in a state-sponsored, board-approved credentialing review. Finally, all physicians will be required to report suspected incompetence, impairment, and drug or alcohol dependence of their colleagues.

The board will create and maintain a clearinghouse for the reports from hospitals, insurers, and physicians. The clearinghouse will also receive reports of any settlements or awards made in the claims resolution process and notifications that disciplinary actions have been taken by other states.[47] The board will review a physician's clearinghouse file whenever it receives one of the required reports.

Unlike many of the present licensing boards, which are generally physician dominated, the Medical Practices Review Board membership will have a minority of physicians. It will also have a full-time staff, which will enable it to carry out investigations of substandard performance. Investigations will be initiated on the basis of adverse reports received by the clearinghouse or complaints about physician performance filed by any member of the public, including board members, hearing examiners who review malpractice claims, and other health care professionals. If there is reason to believe that the physician poses a threat to patient health, the agency will conduct an on-site review and audit of that physician's practices.

When appropriate, board investigators who conduct the required reviews of the clearinghouse files and investigate complaints will recommend that action be taken against a physician by the board's general counsel. The general counsel will then decide whether to initiate a disciplinary charge. If there is evidence of alcoholism, alcohol abuse, drug abuse, or mental illness, the agency will recommend referral to an impaired physician program,[48] regardless of any recommendation to the general counsel on further action. Once a disciplinary charge is initiated, an attorney from the general counsel's office will prosecute the charge before a hearing examiner, who will decide, after a full due-process proceeding, what action, if any, is appropriate. The board's primary mission in such cases is to rehabilitate or reeducate the physician whose practice has become substandard. In cases in which such efforts will not or do not succeed, punitive measures will be imposed, ranging from fines to restrictions on a physician's practices to revocation of the physician's medical license. The examiner's action is subject to review by the board, which will in turn provide notice of any disciplinary action to credentialing entities, insurers, and the medical boards of other states.

To enhance the quality of medical practice, the proposal also requires all physicians to complete at least 50 credit hours of continuing medical education each year. At least 30 of those hours must be directly relevant to the physician's clinical practice. In addition, all physicians will be required to participate in a risk management program.

All of the foregoing physician monitoring and quality assurance requirements and mechanisms are designed to improve the quality of medical care and to reduce medical negligence. Thus, the Project's proposal is a comprehensive response to the medical liability problem.

IMPLICATIONS OF THE PROPOSAL FOR LIABILITY AND ACCESS PROBLEMS

It is widely recognized that the liability crisis in obstetrics plays an important role in the overall liability crisis in medical care.[49] Furthermore, there is no realistic prospect that the liability problems associated with impaired infants will decrease in the future. Under wrongful birth and wrongful life theories of liability, the courts have recently set precedents broadening the physician's legal obligation to diagnose and address foreseeable or potentially recurrent genetic, teratogenic, or chromosomal disorders.[50] From the scientific perspective, current techniques such as electronic fetal monitoring may have enhanced diagnostic ability, but at the same time they have introduced new risks to the fetus.[51] Advances in technology will continue to increase the number of cases in which problematic pregnancies that would otherwise have ended in the death of the fetus result in live but risky births.[52] At the same time, patients' expectations that medicine can guarantee them "perfect" babies will probably continue unabated.[53] The seriousness of the liability crisis in obstetrics calls for careful consideration of dramatically different alternatives. The AMA-Specialty Society proposal is one such alternative.

Before outlining the applicability of the proposal to the obstetrics situation and discussing its implications for that system, a caveat is in order. The discussion focuses primarily on the neurologically impaired infant as the case that poses the greatest difficulty to the current liability system and that most threatens the affordability and availability of maternal and child health care. Many of the implications would hold true in other obstetrics and gynecology cases, however, as well as in nonobstetrical and nongynecological cases.

Implications for Resolving Liability Disputes

Under the proposed plan, the greatest potential changes in the long-term ob-gyn liability situation would come from placing all malpractice claims in an administrative system for resolution. The Project expects adoption of its proposal to lead to the following results.

1. Greater predictability of outcome and awards from experienced, expert decision makers. Predictability and consistency will also be enhanced by having written decisions.[54] Settlements will be encouraged because of the greater certainty about the value of a claim. There should also be some lowering of premiums owing to greater certainty about how claims will be resolved.[55]

2. More accurate evaluation of both negligence and causation by sophisticated, experienced, professional decision makers. By and large, this type of assessment will benefit obstetricians, who now may be found liable whenever there is apparent negligence in the treatment setting, even if the negligence is not causally related to the injury. (In some cases, a more accurate assessment of negligence and causation may lead to findings of liability under the AMA-Specialty Society system where none would be found in the civil jury system. It is highly likely, however, that in such cases the physician will be found responsible for only a small percentage of the injury and therefore only a small percentage of the damage award.) Overall, the Project believes that more accurate determinations of negligence and causation will lead to more accurate allocation of liability, fairer compensation, and greater predictability.[56]

3. Swifter resolution of cases. The mechanisms that encourage settlement under the AMA-Specialty Society system should lead to faster resolution of claims, thereby saving time and money for patients and physicians. Moreover, the administrative system is more streamlined than the courts and is designed to ensure a faster resolution of those cases that remain contested.[57]

4. Lower awards from dispassionate, experienced decision makers. There is no guarantee that this will occur, but common sense suggests that a repeat decision maker will be less swayed by the purely emotional appeal of these cases. Moreover, there may be some lowering of awards because of the requirement that the hearing examiner must identify each specific element of economic damage and explain its basis.

5. Larger number of initial claims. Based on the research of Don Harper Mills[58] and Patricia Danzon,[59] we would expect to see more initial claims filed under the Project's proposal.[60] Claims in which there is no negligence or no causation, however, will be quickly dismissed. Moreover, claims without any out-of-pocket losses by the patient will not

require adjudication, although they may indicate instances where the physician's medical practices warrant attention by the board.

Implications of Proposed Changes in Legal Standards

1. Use of the "prudent and competent practitioner" standard. Use of this modified standard should provide some protection against the imposition of liability for the failure to provide perfect care. In particular, health care providers will have some protection against liability in cases in which they provided the best care possible under circumstances in which specialists or state-of-the-art facilities were unavailable.

2. Slightly stricter rule on qualifications of experts. The modified legal rule governing experts should provide greater assurance of an appropriate assessment of the relevant standard of care.

3. Modification of rules of causation and negligence to "significant contributing factor" and pure comparative negligence. The interaction of these two modified rules will more accurately correlate causation with the obstetrician's liability and will more easily permit the obstetrician to show that a preexisting condition or the mother's own actions (for example, heavy drinking or drug use) contributed to the resulting injury. (The model state statute that is being developed by the Liability Project requires a finding that the health care provider's conduct "increased substantially the risk of an injury and such injury occurred.")

4. Appropriate placement of the burden of proof regarding causation. The civil jury system can lead to a de facto shifting of the burden of proof regarding causation to the defendant. That is, the physician must prove that his deviation from the standard of care did *not* cause the patient's injury.[61] To convince the jury of this, the defendant is effectively required to show that something or someone else definitively caused the injury—a virtual impossibility. Therefore, in the present jury system such cases are often settled even when causation is highly questionable. The clarity of the proposed causation rule in the AMA-Specialty Society's system and its application by a knowledgeable hearing examiner can reasonably be expected to lead to the dismissal of some cases in which liability is currently found due to an erroneous shifting of the burden of proof to the obstetrician.

5. Limitation on noneconomic damages. The proposed variable cap on noneconomic damages will lower total awards and increase their predictability, particularly in jurisdictions that are currently without any limits. (See, for example, the recent $10 million award in an obstetrical malpractice case in Washington, D.C.[62]) However, because the proposal calculates the noneconomic damages cap based on life expectancy, non-

economic damages could still be relatively high for neurologically impaired infants and thus not create any public perception of unfairness.

6. Periodic payment of future damages. The modification of the rule on future damages should ensure that the amounts paid for future damages will more closely correspond to the losses incurred. The requirement of periodic payments for future damages awards in excess of $250,000, coupled with the termination of such payments on the death of the claimant or patient, will lead to a decrease in the total amounts actually paid out in cases in which the claimant is a neurologically impaired infant who does not achieve a normal life expectancy (on which future economic damages are calculated).[63]

7. Establishment of a collateral source rule. The inequity of double recovery by patients will be eliminated by the use of a comprehensive collateral source rule. The application of a collateral source rule to obstetrical negligence awards will lead to potentially great savings for ob-gyns and, through reduced premiums, for ob-gyn patients. The magnitude of the change would be most noticeable in a state that had not already adopted any offset rules.

8. Abolition of joint and several liability. Abolition of the traditional rule of joint and several liability may lead to larger shares of awards being paid by obstetricians in cases in which they are responsible for the larger proportion of the injury. Currently, hospitals may pay a disproportionate share in such cases because they are the "deepest pockets" available to claimants.

Changes Resulting from Improved Physician Monitoring and Credentialing

1. Improvement of the quality of care. This goal of the AMA-Specialty Society proposal is all too often overlooked in discussions of the problems in the medical liability system. The proposed extensive enhancement of physician monitoring activities is designed to lead—and we believe will lead—to higher quality care and fewer instances of medical negligence in obstetrics, as well as in other fields of medicine.

2. Specific changes designed to improve the quality of medical care include

• creation of a centralized state clearinghouse for collecting physician performance data;

• reporting of all settled claims, findings of medical liability, and disciplinary sanctions to the Medical Practices Review Board;

• reporting of all adverse credentialing and all nonclass adverse insurance actions to the board's clearinghouse;

- creation of a professional staff within the agency to investigate disciplinary allegations;
- continuing medical education requirements more closely tailored to the physician's field of practice;
- requirements that performance files be maintained and reviewed on receipt of any adverse report; and
- empowerment of the board to conduct on-site reviews of physician practices, where appropriate.

Possible Modification of the Proposal for Specific Types of Claims

Although the deficiencies of the current system for resolving medical liability disputes are apparent in all fields of medicine, it is in the field of obstetrics that they have received the most scholarly and policymaking attention in recent years. As mentioned earlier, the obvious crisis in obstetrics has led two states, Virginia and Florida, to adopt tort reform proposals directed solely toward the problem of neurologically impaired infants.[64] This situation-specific response raises questions about the suitability of the AMA-Specialty Society proposal as applied to obstetrics or to any other discrete area of medicine.

Through their work with states interested in exploring creative ways of dealing with the crisis in medical liability, Project members have come to recognize that there may be a variety of ways to incorporate aspects of the Project's proposal into an existing state system. Indeed, it is certain that any state considering the AMA-Specialty Society proposal would need to modify the proposal to meet its particular needs. For example, in a state that could ensure adequate funding and professional staffing the disciplinary functions might be performed by the current medical licensing board.

One promising variation of the proposal would be to adopt a scaled-down version for claims arising in obstetrics. Clearly, any state contemplating this variation would have to assess the not insignificant costs of an administrative apparatus against the benefits expected to accrue from fairer, more efficient adjudication of claims involving negligence by obstetricians. Depending on the size of the state, the number of obstetrics claims it handles currently, the extent of the crisis in obstetrics in that state, and the adaptability of its present institutions to the functions called for in the Liability Project proposal, such an experiment might be feasible.

Despite the obvious economies of scale from wholesale adoption of the proposal, there are certain advantages to a more limited experiment. First, a state interested in significant tort reform would be more likely to implement the proposal if it were able to do so initially on a limited basis. The Liability Project is fully aware of and sensitive to legislative reluctance to commit to a far-ranging reform. If a limited application of the proposal to problems in obstetrics will assist in overcoming that natural reluctance, the Project supports its consideration. Second, application of the proposal to a smaller subset of the medical negligence field would provide an extremely useful means of comparing the efficacy of this approach with that of other tort reforms in the field of obstetrics, such as the Virginia and Florida limited no-fault schemes.

Finally, limiting application of the proposal to obstetrics could help determine the extent to which overall problems of access to medical care and availability and affordability of medical malpractice insurance are attributable to obstetrical negligence cases. Given the extraordinarily high potential awards in obstetrical cases (particularly those involving neurologically impaired newborns) and the acknowledged difficulty of proving causation in such cases,[65] it is possible that a limited application of the AMA-Specialty Society proposal to obstetrics would allow awards and insurance rates in other fields of medicine to stabilize.

In light of these possible advantages, the AMA-Specialty Society Project encourages one or more states to consider adopting some type of fault-based, administrative system for adjudicating obstetrical claims, as well as for adjudicating all claims of medical negligence. Although there is no guarantee that the Project's system of claim adjudication and monitoring of physician practices will ameliorate the current crisis in obstetrics, it deserves serious consideration by scholars, legislators, and all persons concerned with ensuring fairer, swifter, and more efficient resolution of medical negligence claims.

In sum the AMA-Specialty Society Medical Liability Project has designed its system with primary attention to fairness—fairness to patients, to physicians, and to the public. We believe that, if our system is implemented on an experimental basis in one or more states, it will be shown to be more equitable than the civil justice system and will improve the quality of and access to medical care for all patients.

REFERENCES AND NOTES

1. A research report prepared by Kendall and Haldi for the U.S. Department of Health, Education, and Welfare found that malpractice insurance premiums for physicians totaled $32 million in 1960, with an additional $29 million being spent by hospitals [Report of the Secretary's Commission on Medical Malpractice. 1973. DHEW Pub. no. (OS) 73-89. Washington, D.C.: Government Printing Office, Appendix 494, p. 509]. According to the U.S. General Accounting Office's 1986 study, Medical Malpractice: Insurance Costs Increased but Varied Among Physicians and Hospitals (GAO/

HRD-86-112, Gaithersburg, Md.), physician premiums in 1985 totaled $3.4 billion (p. 25), with hospital insurance premiums running to $1.34 billion (p. 38).

2. Florida Academic Task Force for Review of the Insurance and Tort Systems. 1987. Preliminary Fact-Finding Report on Medical Malpractice. Gainesville, pp. 152–154 (hereafter referred to as the Florida Academic Task Force).

3. Danzon, P. 1985. Medical Malpractice: Theory, Evidence, and Public Policy. Cambridge, Mass.: Harvard University Press, pp. 59–60. Danzon looks at surveys from 1956 and 1963 that documented 1.3 malpractice claims per 100 physicians annually. St. Paul Fire and Marine Insurance Company, the largest single malpractice carrier, reported a claims rate of 15.4 per 100 physicians (St. Paul's Insurance. 1988. Physicians' and Surgeons' Update. St. Paul. July, p. 1). This claims rate may not fully reflect the crisis in Florida, however, because St. Paul withdrew its malpractice coverage in the state at the end of 1987 (The St. Paul Companies. 1988. Annual Report 1987. St. Paul, pp. 6–7, 46).

4. Georgia Obstetrical and Gynecological Society. 1987. Physician Survey. Atlanta.

5. Medical Association of the State of Alabama. 1988. Survey on Obstetrical Care. Montgomery.

6. University of Colorado Health Sciences Center. 1988. Colorado Obstetrical Care Malpractice Study Report. Denver.

7. American College of Obstetricians and Gynecologists. 1988. Professional Liability and Its Effects: Report of a 1987 Survey of ACOG's Membership. Washington, D.C. The statistics in the text are derived from the survey results.

8. General Accounting Office (GAO), U.S. Congress. 1986. Medical Malpractice: Six State Case Studies Show Claims and Insurance Costs Still Rise Despite Reforms. GAO/HRD-87-21. Gaithersburg, Md. (with few exceptions, the reforms were perceived by the organizations surveyed as having no major impact on the number of claims filed or the size of awards and settlements). Danzon. 1985, pp. 78–79; see note 3 (no discernible effect on claim frequency or severity from virtually all post-1975 tort reforms). See also Sloan, F. 1985. State response to the malpractice insurance "crisis" of the 1970s: An empirical assessment. J. Health Politics Policy Law 9:629–646 (econometric study of the effect of reforms on malpractice premiums found that reforms failed to curb increases in premiums).

9. Tobias, A. 1986. Report of the Twentieth Century Fund Task Force on Medical Malpractice Insurance. Treating Malpractice. New York, p. 6. ("The Task Force does not believe that the current mechanisms for dealing with malpractice do their job.")

10. AFL-CIO Executive Council. 1986. Statement on Liability Insurance and Tort Law. Washington, D.C., p. 3. ("The tort system has contributed to the cost of insurance. . . . In a number of critical respects, the development of new theories of liability and insurer responsibility has led to greater uncertainty in measuring risks.")

11. American Bar Association Action Commission. 1987. Report to Improve the Tort Liability System. Chicago, p. 7. ("[T]here are a host of identifiable problems in tort law that need to be addressed if the system is to function with a greater degree of fairness and efficiency.")

12. New York Governor's Advisory Commission on Liability Insurance. 1986. Insuring Our Future. New York, p. 14. ("[U]nless there are important changes in the liability law that governs the cost of liability protection, this cost . . . will continue to rise at a rapid rate.")

13. After studying the situation in medical malpractice, the GAO concluded that "[a]lternative dispute resolution mechanisms may offer the potential for resolving claims in a more efficient, timely, and equitable manner." General Accounting Office (GAO),

U.S. Congress. 1987. Medical Malpractice: A Framework for Action. GAO/HRD-87-73. Gaithersburg, Md.

14. The Tort Policy Working Group is an interagency group with representatives from 10 federal agencies and the White House. After studying the explosive increase in the number and size of tort awards, particularly medical malpractice awards, the Working Group concluded that the "excesses of the tort system" have contributed significantly to the crisis in insurance availability and affordability. In response they called for a series of tort reforms, including the use of noncourt dispute resolution alternatives, to "bring a greater degree of rationality and predictability to tort law. . . . " Tort Policy Working Group. 1986. Report on the Causes, Extent and Policy Implications of the Current Crisis in Insurance Availability and Affordability. 1986-491-510:40094. Washington, D.C.: Government Printing Office, p. 60.

15. U.S. Department of Health and Human Services. 1987. Report of the Task Force on Medical Liability and Malpractice. Washington, D.C.: Government Printing Office, p. 43. ("Dissatisfaction with the present negligence-based tort system is widespread.")

16. One of the most respected scholars in torts has observed that

   The determination in a malpractice case of a health care provider's fault requires complex and unpredictable litigation which attempts to unravel the often largely unknown mysteries of causation of injury and illness and to determine the appropriateness of treatment procedures about which even experts are often bitterly divided. The process is lengthy, and the results are erratic. Some injured patients recover nothing. Some receive less than fair compensation, some recover amounts far in excess of their actual losses. Large portions of the awards depend on subjective and emotional considerations. The results are often fortuitous, yet society pays high costs for operating this unsatisfactory lottery.

   O'Connell, J. 1984. The case against the current malpractice system. Paper presented at the National Medical Malpractice Conference. February 21. See also Sugarman, R. 1985. Doing away with tort law. Calif. Law Rev. 73:555.

17. Virginia Birth-Related Neurological Injury Compensation Act of 1987, Va. Code Ann. §§ 38.2-5001 to 38.2-5021 (Supp. 1988); Florida Birth-Related Neurological Injury Compensation Plan, 1988 Fla. Sess. Law Serv. ch. 88-1, §§70–75 (West).

18. See, for example, O'Connell, J. 1986. Neo-no-fault remedies for medical injuries: Coordinated statutory and contractual alternatives. Law Contemp. Prob. 49:125.

19. See, for example, the discussion by Richard Epstein in this volume and Epstein, R. 1976. Medical malpractice: The case for contract. Am. Bar Found. Res. J. 76:87.

20. Danzon. 1985, p. 25; see note 3 (study of injuries and claims in California showed that, at most, 1 in 10 malpractice occurrences becomes a claim and that, at most, 1 in 25 patients received compensation). The problem is particularly acute for small claims, for which the high litigation costs more than outweigh any likely recovery. See Tobias. 1986, p. 5; note 9. ("[B]ecause of the staggering costs of trials, many legitimate claims are never brought simply because they are not financially rewarding enough to attract a lawyer.")

21. Moore, W. H., and J. O'Connell. 1984. Foreclosing medical malpractice claims by prompt tender of economic loss. La. Law Rev. 44:1267, 1269 (current system causes similarly situated patients to get varying awards—the result is akin to a lottery). There is also evidence to suggest that, as a group, individuals who sustain injuries as a result of medical negligence receive much higher awards from injuries than do individuals who sustain equivalent injuries in other tort contexts. Chin, A., and M. Peterson. 1985. Deep Pockets, Empty Pockets: Who Wins in Cook County Jury Trials. Santa Monica, Calif.: Rand Corp., p. 55 (average medical malpractice award was five

times the size of jury award for similarly situated personal injury plaintiff and almost twice the size of average award in products liability cases for similar injuries).

22. Tancredi, L. 1986. Compensating for medical injuries: Is there an effective alternative to the tort system of medical malpractice? N. Y. State J. Med. 1986:370, 372 (important defect in tort system is jury's inability to evaluate medical responsibility). Richardson, D., A. Rosoff, and J. McMenamin. 1985. Referral practices and health care costs: The dilemma of high-risk obstetrics. J. Legal Med. 6:427, 443.

23. As discussed earlier, substantial numbers of obstetrician-gynecologists and family practitioners are discontinuing obstetrics practice in response to the rapidly escalating size of obstetrical malpractice awards and the concomitant rise in malpractice insurance premiums. For example, surveys in Arizona and Washington State show that 37 to 40 percent of family practitioners have either stopped or intend to stop their obstetrics practice. Rosenblatt, R. A., and C. L. Wright. 1987. Rising malpractice premiums and obstetric practice patterns. Western J. Med. 146:246–248; Ver Berkmoes, R. 1987. High premiums force Arizona MDs to give up delivering babies. Am. Med. News 30:1. There is also evidence that access to health care may be restricted by physicians' fears of malpractice liability, which cause them to refuse to see certain patients. Charles, S. C., J. R. Wilbert, and K. J. Franke. 1985. Sued and nonsued physicians' self-reported reactions to malpractice litigation. Am. J. Psychiat. 142:437, 440.

24. Sugarman. 1985, p. 596; see note 16. Various estimates report that claimants receive from 18 to 54 percent of each dollar of liability insurance premiums. U.S. Department of Health and Human Services. 1987, p. 16; see note 15.

25. The monies received by the patient are substantially reduced by litigation expenses, including attorneys' fees (usually a one-third contingent fee) and fees for expert witnesses. Gellhorn, E. 1988. Medical malpractice litigation (U.S.)—Medical mishap compensation (N.Z.). Cornell Law Rev. 73:170, 172, note 6.

26. For example, a report on conditions in New Jersey says that the lack of resources and use of part-time board members makes the state medical licensing board ineffective in regulating physicians' competence and quality of care. State of New Jersey Commission of Investigation. 1987. Report and Recommendations on Impaired and Incompetent Physicians. Trenton, pp. 3, 42–43, 74. See also the statement of Kusserow, R. P. 1986. Health Care Quality Improvement Act of 1986: Hearings on H.R. 5540 before the Subcommittee on Civil and Constitutional Rights of the House Committee on the Judiciary. 99th Cong., 2d Sess. 32, 36–37 (Kusserow is inspector general of the U.S. Department of Health and Human Services).

27. O'Connell, J. 1975. No-fault insurance for injuries arising from medical treatment: A proposal for elective coverage. Emory Law J. 24:21.

28. Tancredi, L. 1986. Designing a no-fault alternative. Law Contemp. Prob. 49:277, 281; American Bar Association, Commission on Medical Professional Liability. 1980. Designated Compensable Event System: A Feasibility Study. Chicago, pp. 9–11.

29. Danzon. 1985, pp. 207–218; see note 3. Calabresi, G. 1978. The problem of malpractice: Trying to round out the circle. Pp. 233 and 239 in The Economics of Medical Malpractice, S. Rottenberg, ed. Washington, D.C.: American Enterprise Institute; Epstein, R. 1978. Medical malpractice: Its cause and cure. Pp. 245, 260–262 in The Economics of Medical Malpractice.

30. In 1974 New Zealand abolished medical malpractice litigation and provided a compensation system for personal injury accidents and medical misadventures. Gellhorn. 1988, pp. 170, 188–202; see note 25.

31. On the basis of experience with workers' compensation systems, current commentators have concluded that limited benefits have inadequately compensated the injured

for their full economic loss. Soble, S. M. 1977. A proposal for the administrative compensation of victims of toxic substance pollution: A model act. Harvard J. Legis. 14:683, 715, 717, note 11.

32. Robinson, G. 1986. Rethinking the allocation of medical malpractice risks between patients and providers. Law Contemp. Prob. 49:173, 186–193; see also Zeckhauser, R., and A. Nichols. 1978. Lessons from the economics of safety. Pp. 19, 22, note 7 in The Economics of Medical Malpractice, S. Rottenberg, ed. Washington, D.C.: American Enterprise Institute (communication and interpretation of medical risk information is too limited and difficult to assure patients of fair and efficient contracts).
33. O'Connell. 1986, pp. 125, 137; see note 18.
34. Ibid.
35. Weiler, P., Harvard University. 1988. Legal policy for medical injuries: The issues, the options and the evidence. Unpublished manuscript.
36. Danzon. 1985; see note 3. Tobias. 1986; see note 9.
37. Whether an injury becomes a claim depends to a great extent on factors other than whether the physician is culpable: for example, the severity of a patient's injury or the personal relationship between the physician and patient. Weiler. 1988; see note 35.
38. See, for example, Tancredi. 1986; note 22.
39. See, for example, S. 1804, 99th Cong., 1st Sess., 131 Cong. Rec. 14, 356–359 (1985); H.R. 3084, 99th Cong., 1st Sess., 131 Cong. Rec. 6353 (1985).
40. See the Report of the Committee on Administrative Procedure. S. 8, 77th Cong., 1st Sess. 30 (1941) (reasons for requiring an opinion are guidance for future conduct and parties' satisfaction with result).
41. Louisell, D., and H. Williams. 1988. Medical Malpractice. New York: Matthew Bender, 8.04 (traditional standard of care is based on the custom of the locality).
42. The standard of care is not wholly objective and "mere differences of methods do not imply deviation from the standard of care if it appears that each method can reasonably be regarded as acceptable." Ibid., 8.57.
43. Ibid., 8.07.
44. Ibid., 22.06.
45. The workers' compensation schemes were also designed in part to promote the efficient resolution of claims. Architects of these state systems have recognized that consistent decision making is "an important factor in reducing the frequency of litigation" and inducing settlement. Prototype of an Administrative Workers' Compensation System. 1982. Camp Hill, Pa.: American Insurance Association, p. 44.
46. Nonmarket mechanisms, such as licensing and education, may be necessary to ensure competent and quality health care. Shavell, S. 1978. Theoretical issues in medical malpractice. Pp. 35, 49, 55 in The Economics of Medical Malpractice, S. Rottenberg, ed. Washington, D.C.: American Enterprise Institute.
47. Much of this information will already be reported to a centralized clearinghouse established by recent federal legislation. Federal Health Care Quality Improvement Act of 1986, 42 U.S.C. §§ 11101-52 (Supp. 1988). Since November 14, 1987, all medical malpractice insurers must report all payments on lawsuits or claims to the secretary of the Department of Health and Human Services and to the appropriate licensing board in the state in which the action arose [ibid., § 11131(b)]. Failure to comply results in a maximum penalty of $10,000 for each payment not reported [ibid., § 11131(c)].
48. An impaired physician program is a medically directed treatment program for physicians impaired by alcoholism, alcohol abuse, drug abuse, or mental illness. See, for example, American Medical Association. 1983. AMA's Impaired Physician Program: Report of the Board of Trustees I-83. Chicago.

49. Richardson et al. 1985, pp. 427, 462, note 125; see note 22. ("The stakes are particularly high in perinatal care, since the brain damage or other permanent, incapacitating defects which can result from delivery mishaps make the long-term care of the injured infant an extremely expensive proposition.") American Medical Association—Special Task Force on Professional Liability and Insurance. 1984. Professional Liability in the 80's. Chicago, pp. 8, 19. (In 1984 the midpoint verdict for medical injuries to newborns was $1,452,211, compared with a midpoint verdict in 1983–1984 of $200,637 for suits against physicians generally.)

50. Coplan, J. 1985. Wrongful life and wrongful birth: New concepts for the pediatrician. Pediatrics 75:65.

51. Richardson et al. 1985, pp. 427, 438; see note 22.

52. For example, medical advances have dramatically increased the survival rate of low-birthweight infants, who are typically born prematurely. A baby weighing two pounds at birth now has a 50 percent survival rate, compared with a 6 percent survival rate more than 20 years ago (Dougherty, C. J. 1985. The right to begin life with sound body and mind: Fetal patients and conflicts with their mothers. Univ. Detroit Law Rev. 63:89, 105). Although more low-birthweight babies now survive, such babies often experience significant physical and mental impairments and require costly, long-term care. Hughes, D., K. Johnson, S. Rosenbaum, E. Butler, and J. Simons. 1987. The Health of America's Children: Maternal and Child Health Data Book. Washington, D.C.: Children's Defense Fund, p. 26. See also *Akron v. Akron Center for Reproductive Health,* 462 U.S. 416, 457 (1982).

53. Stratton, W. 1987. Birth defect suits: The cost. Kan. Med. 88:320; Tobias. 1986, p. 29; see note 9 (causes of the growing number of medical malpractice claims include greater patient expectations).

54. The current jury system produces much uncertainty because juries are not required to articulate reasons for awards and thus their decisions cannot be scrutinized by insurers, lawyers, and claimants to establish reliable predictions for future claims. Trebilcock, M. 1986. The insurance deterrence dilemma of modern tort law. Paper presented at the National Conference of State Legislatures seminar: Controlling Liability Costs. State Actions and Alternatives. New Orleans, December 14–16.

55. Iglehart, J. 1986. The professional liability crisis: The 1986 Duke private sector conference. N. Eng. J. Med. 315:1105, 1106 (according to Jeffrey O'Connell, one of insurers' principal concerns is uncertainty in the tort system).

56. Arbiters who repeatedly hear complex medical claims have developed a better understanding of the scientific evidence as their knowledge of medical care issues has increased (Tancredi. 1986, pp. 370, 373; see note 22). Historically, one principal justification for establishing an administrative agency has been "the need to bring to bear upon particular problems technical or professional skills." Specialists may hone these skills through recurring agency work (Report of the Committee on Administrative Procedure. 1941; see note 40). See also Stein, J., G., Mitchell, and B. Mezines. 1988. Medical Malpractice. New York: Matthew Bender § 1.01[2].

57. The efficiency of the traditional court system can be improved. One often-cited estimate is that jury trials consume 40 percent more time than bench trials (Zeisel, H., H. Kalven, Jr., and B. Buchholz. 1959. Delay in the Court. Boston: Little, Brown, pp. 71–81). According to one study, an arbitration system decreased the amount of time for processing a claim in the court system by 13 percent (Tancredi. 1986, p. 373; see note 22). Similarly, workers' compensation hearing officers can decide claims more quickly because they are more familiar with the medical terminology and the law (Prototype of an Administrative Workers' Compensation System. 1982; see note 45).

58. In his classic study of hospital records in California, Mills found a surprisingly large number of injuries caused by negligent medical treatment (Mills, D. H. 1977. Medical Insurance Feasibility Study. San Francisco: Sutter).

59. Danzon. 1985; see note 3.

60. Because the current system generates claims for fewer than 20 percent of the actual malpractice incidents detected in medical records, an administrative proposal removing the barriers to access to the system should result in a larger number of initial claims (see Schwartz, W., and N. Komesar. 1978. Doctors, damages, and deterrence: An economic view of medical malpractice. N. Eng. J. Med. 298:1282, 1286).

61. The complex medical and causation issues that are involved result in the expansion of the concept of negligence; thus, defendants are functionally held strictly liable for medical injuries (Trebilcock. 1986; see note 54).

62. See Hockstader, L. 1988. Boy gets $10 million for birth defect; Judgment against 3 doctors one of the largest in the area. Washington Post. May 14, p. B-1.

63. Periodic payment awards also help ensure the real future purchasing power intended by the decision maker because the insurer can hedge inflation with an indexed annuity. Thus, the market and not the jury discounts the awards. The cost will be minimized because the insurer can seek the cheapest annuities in the market (Danzon. 1985, pp. 164–165; see note 3).

64. Danzon. 1985, p. 8 and note 19; see (reference) note 3.

65. See, for example, the recent data suggesting that it may be difficult to distinguish infant brain damage caused by improper obstetrical care from infant brain damage caused by maternal use of cocaine (Brody, J. E. 1988. Cocaine: Litany of fetal risks grows. New York Times [Chicago ed.]. September 6, p. 19).

The Shadow of the Law: Jury Decisions in Obstetrics and Gynecology Cases*

STEPHEN DANIELS, PH.D., AND LORI ANDREWS, J.D.

In his address to the 52nd annual meeting of the Central Association of Obstetricians and Gynecologists in 1984, Kenneth J. Vander Kolk took as his theme the title of the Peggy Lee song, "Is That All There Is?" He told his colleagues that "we practice in a cage of sorts, the bars of which are made from an alloy of legal scrutiny, legal harassment, legal endeavors, some legal expertise, and a good portion of legal omnipotence."[1] Physicians, he claimed, "are an easy prey for the hustling attorney who initiates a lawsuit."[2] Using 1954 as a point of comparison, Vander Kolk bemoaned the loss of innocence of an earlier time when an obstetrician-gynecologist's cost of business (including liability insurance) was so much lower. "There was practically no malpractice. There was no Medicaid, no Medicare, no health maintenance organizations, no preferred provider organizations, no diagnosis-related groups, and most patients paid in cash. These were the good old days, but were they really any better?"[3]

At least in terms of medical malpractice, Vander Kolk, like many of his colleagues, thinks things are far worse today than in the good old

* The research reported in this chapter was supported in part by a grant from the National Foundation, Law and Social Sciences Program, Grant no. SES87-09794. The authors would like to thank Ami Jaeger, Ruth Sosniak, Leah Feldman, and Lorrie Wessel for their help in the preparation of this paper, and Rebecca Wilkin for her expert supervision of the data collection.

days. In his view, "no longer can anything less than a perfect result in patient care be considered to be an act of God, as it was in 1954."[4] Although it is unlikely that he would use the reference, Vander Kolk's viewpoint with regard to malpractice—and one with which many of his colleagues might agree—can be nicely summed up in the title of a more recent song, one by the Grateful Dead: things are going to "Hell in a Bucket."[5]

Vander Kolk's characterization of medical malpractice echoes that of many other physicians, their professional organizations, and the companies that sell liability insurance to them. As Harold Schulman described it in his presidential address to the New York Obstetrical Society, "Malpractice litigation has profoundly influenced our professional lives. It has become the single most talked about topic among physicians."[6]

In 1985 William Mixson, then president of the American College of Obstetricians and Gynecologists, said that malpractice was the most serious problem facing obstetricians and gynecologists.[7] The same conclusion was reached by the American Medical Association's Obstetrics-Gynecology Council on Long-Range Planning and Development: "This crisis is perhaps the most potent environmental factor currently affecting obstetricians and gynecologists."[8]

Although many medical commentators concede that malpractice does occur, the majority attack the tort system as a means of handling the problem. Often, there are the expected derogatory claims about lawyers. As Vander Kolk puts it, "will the unlimited classes of graduating lawyers increase the number involved in unbridled, insensitive, inconsiderate, and unethical litigation?"[9] More typical are charges about what actually happens when a malpractice matter enters the courts. In particular it is argued that juries are not deciding the cases rationally.[10] According to Otis Bowen, former secretary of the Department of Health and Human Services, "It has become more a lottery than a rational system for compensation to the injured."[11] The damages awarded are criticized as being overly generous.[12]

In addition, some commentators suggest that the errors providing the basis for malpractice suits cannot easily be avoided. For example, American Medical Association (AMA) counsel Kirk Johnson points out that medicine "requires decisions that are often as much matters of judgment as of science."[13] Other commentators suggest that sophisticated new technologies are the basis for suits. AMA executive vice-president James Sammons, for example, suggested that errors may be due to "highly advanced but imperfect technology."[14] The implication is that juries may be unfairly holding physicians liable for maloccurrences that are not easily preventable. Along those lines, Bowen pointed out that physicians feel that they are "unfairly at risk of being sued."[15]

AMA counsel Johnson has said that it is "the unpredictability of the system—the vagaries of juries and the uncertainty about what is 'fault' and when fault 'causes' harm to an already ill or injured patient—that makes it hard for physicians to know what is 'legal' negligence and substantially undercuts the system's deterrent effect."[16] In his view, "there are wide, irrational variations in both findings of liability and the amount of damages for similar cases."[17]

Despite the fact that jury verdicts in medical malpractice cases are roundly criticized, there have been surprisingly few studies of what actually happens in malpractice cases that go to court and virtually no studies of cases involving obstetricians and gynecologists. Previous studies have addressed malpractice jury verdicts only peripherally.[18] There has been more direct analysis of malpractice insurance claims, most prominently Patricia Danzon's research[19] and the recent U.S. General Accounting Office studies.[20] Based on the findings of the studies to date, however, the connection between the problems faced by physicians and what happens to malpractice disputes in the legal system remains an open question.

In this chapter we report on a study that focused exclusively on medical malpractice jury awards; our discussion here emphasizes obstetrics and gynecology cases. The study was based on an analysis of data from all medical malpractice jury verdicts in 46 counties in 11 states from 1981 to 1985. Although only a small percentage of claims against physicians proceeds all the way to a jury decision, the actions of juries influence the amount of compensation insurance companies will pay on similar claims settled out of court. In addition, assumptions about jury verdicts have been used to justify many recent tort reform proposals.

We examine the quantity and nature of malpractice jury verdicts against a backdrop of the potential claims patients have against physicians. In doing this we will use two metaphors: a pyramid and a shadow. The pyramid is used to place malpractice jury verdicts in the broader context of disputes between physicians and patients by illustrating how few medical errors that cause patient injury actually result in a jury trial. Jury verdicts are at the pinnacle of the pyramid.

The shadow shows the broader importance of jury verdicts: despite their small numbers, they cast a large shadow down the sides of the pyramid. Estimates suggest that about 90 percent of all civil disputes are settled without a trial, through a process of negotiation. Because of the potential for resorting to legal action, however, negotiation is based on the likely decision of the courts. Thus, negotiation takes place—in the words of a number of commentators—in the "shadow of the law."[21] It is the familiar image of a small object casting a disproportionately large shadow.

We describe the shadow cast by obstetrics and gynecology cases by focusing on a series of questions about what actually happens when these cases go to a jury: What types of obstetrics and gynecology cases go to a jury? How severe are the alleged injuries? What is the nature of those injuries? What is the alleged cause of the injury? Who wins? When plaintiffs win, how much do they win?

The accepted wisdom blames the legal system for the problems faced by doctors. Physicians and commentators have argued that there are too many lawsuits, too many jury awards for plaintiffs, and too many large awards made in an unpredictable fashion. In contrast, we find that few of these cases go before a jury, that plaintiffs do not usually win, and that there are identifiable patterns in what juries decide in the cases that come before them.

JURY VERDICTS AND THE DISPUTE RESOLUTION PYRAMID

A useful way to visualize the generation and resolution of disputes between patients and physicians is to view the process as a pyramid. At the base of the pyramid is the universe of medical events that have the potential for generating disputes between patients and their physicians. These are the medical errors resulting in injury that could provide the basis for a claim by the patient against the physician. As with other types of legal disputes,[22] only a few of the many potential malpractice disputes go all the way from the base to the top of the pyramid. At the pinnacle are those few issues resolved by jury trial. The pyramid is oddly shaped, with a broad base and relatively flat sides.

With respect to obstetrics and gynecology (and medical treatment more generally), the precise dimensions of the pyramid are unknown. Each time a health care professional comes into contact with a patient or makes a decision regarding a patient's care, the chance of error arises. There is probably no way of finding out the actual number of medical errors committed in the course of treatment, and the paucity of reliable data limits what can be said about the remainder of the pyramid.

Relying on the available data, we can provide a rough outline of this pyramid's shape. We draw on studies in the medical literature and in the insurance claims literature for estimates of the amount of medical error causing patient injury and the resulting number of patient claims against health care professionals. These estimates are supplemented by estimates of errors and claims we have made using figures on hospital admissions available from federal sources and sources in Texas (one of the states in our study of jury verdicts). To provide some idea of how many medical errors eventually lead to a court filing and then to an actual trial, we rely on figures from New York (another state in our study).

It appears that the absolute amount of error is likely to be substantial. For instance, an influential study of the quality of medical care by Brook and Stevenson found that only 27 percent of the emergency room patients in a major city hospital received effective care; 60 percent received ineffective care, and 13 percent received neither effective nor ineffective care.[23] Brook and colleagues repeated the study at the Johns Hopkins Hospital, focusing on patients complaining of gastrointestinal symptoms. They found that only 25 percent were given acceptable care.[24]

Consistent with such findings, Patricia Danzon's study of malpractice insurance claims[25] suggests that, on average, 1 in 20 hospital patients incurs an injury as a result of medical error. Danzon based her estimates on an earlier California Medical Association (CMA) and California Hospital Association (CHA) study;[26] these estimates, she says, probably understate the true rate.[27] Using her formula and readily available statistics, we can calculate a rough, conservative estimate of the universe of medical error resulting in patient injury. The National Center for Health Statistics reports that 34.3 million patients (excluding newborn infants) were discharged from short-stay, nonfederal hospitals in 1986.[28] Using Danzon's 1 in 20 formula, the estimate of the universe of medical error resulting in patient injury in the United States in 1986 was at least 1,715,000.

We can provide some detail on this aggregate estimate of medical error by moving to the state level. Looking at Texas, we find that, in 1983, 2.5 million people were admitted to short-term general hospitals.[29] Using Danzon's 1 in 20 estimate of errors resulting in injuries for hospital admissions, the universe of medical error in Texas for 1983 should have been in the neighborhood of 125,000. The universe of error resulting in injury in the obstetrics and gynecology area will also be sizable. For instance, we can calculate a rough estimate of the amount of error in Texas with respect to labor and delivery by using Danzon's 1 in 20 estimate and the number of live births. In 1983 in Texas there were 295,000 live births,[30] potentially representing an estimated 14,750 errors resulting in injury.

There have been few attempts to discern why and how particular medical errors are transformed into claims by patients against physicians. What we do know suggests that most errors resulting in patient injury do not lead to malpractice claims. For instance, the CMA and CHA asked panels of medical and legal experts to examine 20,864 inpatient charts from 23 hospitals in California to identify potentially compensable injuries.[31] They found some evidence of fault in 17 percent of the charts.[32] They also found that only about 10 percent of those patients actually filed a claim. A similar finding emerges from Danzon's nationwide analysis of the frequency and severity of malpractice insurance claims against doctors and hospitals.[33] She found that few instances of injury caused by medical error led to an insurance claim. She reports that "at most 1 in 10 negligent injuries resulted in a claim, and of these 40 percent received payment. In other words, at most 1 in 25 negligent injuries [sic] result in compensation through the malpractice system."[34]

If we return to the data for Texas, we find even lower claims rates. Using Danzon's formula of 1 in 10 injured patients making claims against health care professionals, we would expect a total of about 12,600 malpractice claims for 1983 (corresponding to the estimated 126,000 errors resulting in patient injuries) and about 1,470 claims dealing with labor and delivery (corresponding to the estimate of 14,750 errors resulting in patient injuries). The actual claims rates were much lower. A Texas State Board of Medical Examiners report shows that 1,701 malpractice claims were made in 1983, of which only 219 were for *all* obstetrics and gynecology matters.[35] An earlier report shows that between 1978 and 1984 there were only 1,178 obstetrics and gynecology claims filed in Texas.[36]

Like the California figures, these low rates for Texas strongly suggest that most patients who are injured by medical error will not pursue a claim. Only one study to date has investigated the dynamics of dispute transformation at this level. May and DeMarco surveyed patients in two southern Wisconsin communities who were dissatisfied with the medical care they received. They found that the most common responses to patient dissatisfaction were to "lump it" (do nothing) or simply to change doctors. Only 25 percent of the patients contacted the offending physician directly, and only 11 percent contacted a lawyer.[37]

Patients who do pursue claims against physicians do not always collect from the insurers. The great majority of claims, whether malpractice claims generally or obstetrics and gynecology claims specifically, are settled out of court, with or without payment—at a rate of about 90 percent. Furthermore, according to Danzon, only about 50 percent of these are likely to be settled with a payment. Similarly, a national study by the National Association of Insurance Commissioners found that only 46 percent of malpractice insurance claims were settled with a payment.[38] In Texas only 21 percent of the obstetrics and gynecology claims were settled with a payment; for all malpractice claims, the figure was 20.3 percent.[39] Using these scattered examples, we begin to see the dispute resolution pyramid taking shape.

The sides of the pyramid grow no steeper when we look at court filings for malpractice suits. Unfortunately, little is known about the actual number of obstetrics and gynecology court filings for malpractice, so we are left to draw a rough estimate of the situation. Only a few state court systems keep detailed enough statistics to tell the number of medical malpractice filings generally, and none breaks the figures down further. New York is one state that reports overall medical malpractice court filings. Looking at three New York counties in our study, for instance, we find that in 1984 there were 476 medical malpractice cases filed in Kings County, 490 filed in New York County, and 35 filed in upstate Monroe County, which includes Rochester (data provided by State of New York, Office of Court Administration, 1988).

Surely, there were more medical errors and more malpractice claims than court filings in these three counties. Using Danzon's 1 in 20 estimate for errors per hospital admission causing patient injury and 1984 hospital admission data from the American Hospital Association's annual survey[40] along with these court filing data, we calculate the following rough estimates of medical errors resulting in injuries for these counties in 1984: Kings, 12,353 (247,055 admissions); Monroe, 4,104 (82,085 admissions); and New York, 23,723 (474,468 admissions). In terms of the ratio of estimated error to actual court filings for these counties in 1984, we find the following: Kings, 1 malpractice filing per 26 hospital admissions; New York, 1 per 48 admissions; and Monroe, 1 per 117 admissions. These figures illustrate that there are far fewer malpractice court filings than errors resulting in injury.

The New York State filing statistics for these counties provide another piece of important information: how the filed malpractice cases were disposed of by the trial courts. Few of the cases—generally speaking, fewer than 18 percent—actually went to a jury trial. At least 70 percent were settled or stricken from the docket, and the remainder were handled in a variety of other ways. There is no reason to assume that the picture is significantly different for the subset of malpractice cases that involves obstetrics and gynecology.

Only a small proportion of the substantial number of medical errors resulting in patient injuries are transformed into claims, and no more than one-half of those that are transformed are settled with a payment. The great bulk of claims are settled out of court, and most that go as far as a court filing never go to trial.

JURY VERDICTS AND THE SHADOW THEY CAST

The importance of jury verdicts lies not in their numbers, but in their symbolic value as "transmitters of signals rather than as deciders of cases."[41] They play a crucial role in setting the "going rates" for different

TABLE 1   Selected Sites and Total Number of Civil Jury Verdicts

County	Court	Years	No. of Verdicts
Maricopa, Ariz.	Superior	1981–1985	1,765
Alameda, Calif.	Superior	1981–1985	357
Fresno, Calif.	Superior	1981–1985	157
Los Angeles, Calif.	Superior	1981–1985	2,613
Sacramento, Calif.	Superior	1981–1985	509
San Diego, Calif.	Superior	1981–1985	410
San Francisco, Calif.	Superior	1981–1985	668
Arapahoe, Colo.	District	1984–1985	51
Boulder, Colo.	District	1984–1985	53
Denver, Colo.	District	1984–1985	294
Jefferson, Colo.	District	1984–1985	94
Cobb, Ga.	Superior	1982–1984	90
DeKalb, Ga.	Superior	1982–1984	239
Fulton, Ga.	Superior	1982–1984	539
Cook, Ill.	Circuit	1981–1985	4,181
DuPage, Ill.	Circuit	1981–1985	436
Kane, Ill.	Circuit	1981–1985	171
Lake, Ill.	Circuit	1981–1985	295
McHenry, Ill.	Circuit	1981–1985	61
Will, Ill.	Circuit	1981–1985	290
Winnebago, Ill.	Circuit	1981–1985	148
Johnson, Kan.	District	1981–1985	310
Wyandotte, Kan.	District	1981–1985	286
Clay, Mo.	Circuit	1981–1985	104
Jackson, Mo.	Circuit	1981–1985	894
Platte, Mo.	Circuit	1981–1985	47
Bronx, N.Y.	Supreme	1981–1985	367
Erie, N.Y.	Supreme	1983–1985	181
Kings, N.Y.	Supreme	1981–1985	762
Monroe, N.Y.	Supreme	1983–1985	127
Nassau, N.Y.	Supreme	1981–1985	636
New York, N.Y.	Supreme	1981–1985	1,101
Onondaga, N.Y.	Supreme	1983–1985	86
Queens, N.Y.	Supreme	1981–1985	404
Richmond, N.Y.	Supreme	1981–1985	71
Suffolk, N.Y.	Supreme	1981–1985	291
Westchester, N.Y.	Supreme	1981–1985	259
Multnomah, Ore.	Circuit	1984–1985	285
Dallas, Tex.	District	1981–1985	2,106
Harris, Tex.	District	1981–1985	2,012
King, Wash.	Superior	1983–1985	416
Pierce, Wash.	Superior	1983–1985	131
Skagit, Wash.	Superior	1983–1985	19

TABLE 1 *continued*

County	Court	Years	No. of Verdicts
Snohomish, Wash.	Superior	1983–1985	114
Spokane, Wash.	Superior	1983–1985	122
Yakima, Wash.	Superior	1983–1985	73
Total			24,625

types of cases, and these going rates in turn are used in the process of negotiation and settlement that disposes of the bulk of claims. Galanter has said that "we might visualize the jury as a part of a system of 'bargaining in the shadow of the law.' The jury casts a shadow across the wider arena of claims and settlements by communication of signals about what future juries might do."[42] The jury's principal contribution "to dispute resolution is providing a background of norms and procedures against which negotiations . . . take place."[43]

We were interested in determining the shape of the shadow cast by medical malpractice jury verdicts over other phases of the dispute process involving medical error. We also wanted to know how this shadow compared with the one cast by civil jury verdicts generally so that we would have some larger context to use in describing malpractice jury shadow. To do this, we first collected data on 24,625 civil verdicts from state trial courts of general jurisdiction in 46 counties in 11 states for the years 1981 to 1985. The sites included in our study, along with the raw frequencies, are given in Table 1. The sites are not a representative sample of all jurisdictions across the country; rather, they reflect a combination of regional balance and available source materials.

The jury verdict data were collected from local jury reporters. These reporters are subscription services used by local attorneys, judges, insurance companies, and so on. The reporters we used are nonselective in their coverage of cases. They do not limit themselves to certain types of cases (e.g., auto accidents) or to those considered important for some reason (e.g., those with high awards). They get their information directly from court records and from the attorneys involved. The case reports published by these services indicate the county in which the jury verdict was rendered; when it was rendered; the names of the parties and the attorneys; the type of case; a short description of the factual situation; the jury's verdict and award, if one was given; apportionment of liability, where appropriate; any special damages; compensatory or general damages; and any punitive, exemplary, or multiplied damages.[44]

For each of the 46 counties in each year, data were collected on *all* published jury cases in which money damages were at issue. The data generally cover the period 1981–1985, although fewer years are covered for some sites because of problems in obtaining data (see Table 1). The data presented here are for all years combined. Combining the data allows us to give an overall picture of patterns in jury verdicts for the first half of the 1980s while controlling for year-to-year fluctuations in verdicts.[45] Moreover, five years is too short a period to use in talking about trends. The data do not include verdicts in federal trials, verdicts in bench trials, settlements short of trial, or posttrial motions.[46] All dollar amounts are presented in 1985 dollars, and jury awards represent gross awards rather than net awards (after reductions for comparative negligence).

From the general jury verdict data set of 24,625 cases, we identified 1,885 (7.7 percent) that involved allegations of medical malpractice. Among these malpractice cases, we identified 364 obstetrics and gynecology cases (19.3 percent of the malpractice cases and 1.5 percent of all the jury cases). We then collected additional data on the obstetrics and gynecology cases (as defined by the nature of treatment involved and not just the physician's specialty). These data are the subject of our analysis.

We first take a broad view of malpractice verdicts. This task involves describing how the 1,885 malpractice verdicts and the 364 obstetrics and gynecology verdicts were distributed among the 46 counties and how often plaintiffs won. We show how the obstetrics and gynecology verdicts were distributed by type of case (pregnancy, tubal ligation, and so on) and look at those verdicts in terms of the severity of injury alleged, the cause of injury, and how much money plaintiffs were awarded when they did win.

Second, we provide more detail, looking at plaintiff success rates, severity of injury, cause of injury, and size of awards for the different types of obstetrics and gynecology cases. Throughout our discussion, we refer to our background data on total civil jury verdicts to provide a context for the information on malpractice verdicts.

JURY VERDICTS IN OBSTETRICS AND GYNECOLOGY

General Contours of the Shadow

Distribution of Verdicts Among Sites

Table 2 presents data on the number of medical malpractice cases in each of the 46 counties, the percentage of all money damage cases accounted for by malpractice, the number of obstetrics and gynecology cases, and the percentage of all malpractice cases involving obstetrics

TABLE 2   Number and Percentage of Medical Malpractice and
Obstetrics-Gynecology (Ob-Gyn) Verdicts in Selected Counties,
1981–1985

County	Medical Malpractice (N)	Medical Malpractice as % of All Verdicts	Ob-Gyn (N)	Ob-Gyn as % of All Medical Malpractice
Maricopa, Ariz.	50	2.8	10	20.0
Alameda, Calif.	32	9.0	5	15.6
Fresno, Calif.	12	7.6	2	16.7
Los Angeles, Calif.	305	11.7	56	18.4
Sacramento, Calif.	27	5.3	4	14.8
San Diego, Calif.	39	9.5	5	12.8
San Francisco, Calif.	38	5.7	4	10.5
Arapahoe, Colo.	3	5.9	1	33.3
Boulder, Colo.	4	7.5	1	25.0
Denver, Colo.	29	9.9	3	10.3
Jefferson, Colo.	10	10.6	1	10.0
Cobb, Ga.	8	8.9	1	12.5
DeKalb, Ga.	17	7.1	0	—
Fulton, Ga.	35	6.5	9	25.7
Cook, Ill.	134	3.2	26	19.4
DuPage, Ill.	28	6.4	5	17.9
Kane, Ill.	10	5.8	2	20.0
Lake, Ill.	19	6.4	4	21.1
McHenry, Ill.	8	13.1	2	25.0
Will, Ill.	22	7.6	3	13.6
Winnebago, Ill.	8	5.4	1	12.5
Johnson, Kan.	17	5.5	4	23.5
Wyandotte, Kan.	10	3.5	2	20.0
Clay, Mo.	4	3.8	0	—
Jackson, Mo.	38	4.3	9	23.7
Platte, Mo.	1	2.1	0	—
Bronx, N.Y.	43	11.7	10	23.3
Erie, N.Y.	17	9.4	6	35.3
Kings, N.Y.	150	19.7	26	17.3
Monroe, N.Y.	5	3.9	0	—
Nassau, N.Y.	121	19.0	33	27.3
New York, N.Y.	224	20.3	43	19.2
Onondaga, N.Y.	9	10.5	4	44.4
Queens, N.Y.	85	21.0	22	25.9
Richmond, N.Y.	10	14.1	5	50.0
Suffolk, N.Y.	36	12.4	11	30.6
Westchester, N.Y.	46	17.8	10	21.7
Multnomah, Ore.	18	6.3	7	38.9
Dallas, Tex.	42	2.0	4	9.5
Harris, Tex.	117	5.8	11	9.4

TABLE 2 *continued*

County	Medical Malpractice (N)	Medical Malpractice as % of All Verdicts	Ob-Gyn (N)	Ob-Gyn as % of All Medical Malpractice
King, Wash.	33	7.9	6	18.2
Pierce, Wash.	7	5.3	3	42.9
Skagit, Wash.	0	—	0	—
Snohomish, Wash.	4	3.5	1	25.0
Spokane, Wash.	4	3.3	0	—
Yakima, Wash.	6	8.2	2	33.3
Total	1,885		364	

and gynecology verdicts. The specific courts involved and the years included for each site can be found in Table 1, together with the total number of verdicts from which the malpractice percentage is calculated.

Perhaps the most notable aspect of Table 2 is the variation among sites in the number of malpractice jury cases. The number ranges from 0 in small Skagit County, Washington, and 1 in Platte County, Missouri, to 305 in Los Angeles County, California (it is important to keep in mind that this is a five-year total for Los Angeles). Table 2 also shows that medical malpractice jury cases were not numerous during the early 1980s. Except for the largest population centers, the number of malpractice jury cases remained below 50. Only six counties had more than 100 malpractice cases for the period: Los Angeles County; Cook County, Illinois; Kings, Nassau, and New York counties in New York; and Harris County, Texas. Generally speaking, malpractice cases did not constitute a large proportion of all jury verdicts. They were 10 percent or more of all jury verdicts in only 12 of the 46 counties, and 9 of those 12 were in New York State.

There was great variation in the number of obstetrics and gynecology cases and in the proportion of malpractice cases accounted for by obstetrics and gynecology verdicts. In the 45 counties with malpractice verdicts (Skagit County had none), the number of obstetrics and gynecology cases ranged from 0 in 5 counties to 56 in Los Angeles County. Only 11 counties had 10 or more obstetrics and gynecology cases in the early 1980s, and 7 of the 11 were in New York State.

In the 40 counties that had them, obstetrics and gynecology cases as a percentage of all malpractice cases ranged from 9.4 percent to 50.0 percent. Obstetrics and gynecology cases generally made up sizable proportions of total malpractice verdicts—indeed, often the largest proportion. In the 22 of the 45 counties with malpractice verdicts, obstetrics and gynecology cases accounted for 20 percent or more of the verdicts. In the larger counties, which had greater numbers of malpractice cases, the percentage was somewhat lower: in the eight counties with 50 or more medical malpractice jury verdicts, the percentage of obstetrics and gynecology cases was 20 percent or lower in all but two, Nassau and Queens counties in New York.

Plaintiff Success Rates

Contrary to what one might expect in light of the rhetoric of malpractice, we found that plaintiffs were not likely to be successful in medical malpractice cases generally or in obstetrics and gynecology cases specifically (success being defined as an award of at least $1). In medical malpractice cases generally, the success rate was 32.4 percent; in obstetrics and gynecology cases it was slightly higher, 36.8 percent. These success rates are in sharp contrast to other types of civil jury cases. When we looked at all civil jury verdicts involving money damages, we found that plaintiffs tended to be successful more often than not, with an overall success rate of 57 percent.[47]

Table 3 presents data on plaintiff success rates for all civil jury verdicts, for medical malpractice jury verdicts, and for obstetrics and gynecology jury verdicts. The overall success rate for each county was calculated from the frequencies in Table 1 (the number of jury verdicts in which the plaintiff was awarded at least $1 divided by the total number of verdicts). The medical malpractice and obstetrics and gynecology success rates were calculated using the frequencies in Table 2.

The success rates for all jury verdicts ranged from 40.2 percent in Westchester County, New York, to 78.9 percent in Skagit County, Washington. Skagit County, however, is a very small jurisdiction with only a handful of jury cases. Most overall success rates (29 of 46) were between 55 and 65 percent.

The picture is quite different when we move to plaintiff success rates for medical malpractice generally. These success rates ranged from 0 in three counties to 75 percent in two counties; these five counties, however, each had no more than four malpractice jury cases. The range narrows in counties with more cases. Success rates for sites with 50 or more malpractice cases (eight counties) range from 10.3 percent to 48.2 percent.

Overall, the highest plaintiff success rates in general malpractice cases were to be found in the New York counties. Four of the sites with 50 or more malpractice cases were in New York, and three of them had success rates of more than 40 percent. Comparing plaintiff success rates for all jury verdicts with those for malpractice cases shows that

TABLE 3   Plaintiff Success Rates in Selected Counties, 1981–1985

County	Overall	Medical Malpractice	Ob-Gyn
Maricopa, Ariz.	58.4	28.0	10.0
Alameda, Calif.	56.0	31.3	20.0
Fresno, Calif.	50.3	8.3	0.0
Los Angeles, Calif.	55.7	30.8	37.5
Sacramento, Calif.	54.2	22.2	0.0
San Diego, Calif.	48.8	41.0	20.0
San Francisco, Calif.	60.0	39.5	25.0
Arapahoe, Colo.	60.8	0.0	0.0
Boulder, Colo.	72.2	0.0	0.0
Denver, Colo.	54.4	20.7	33.3
Jefferson, Colo.	56.4	10.0	0.0
Cobb, Ga.	64.4	12.5	0.0
DeKalb, Ga.	58.2	11.8	—
Fulton, Ga.	58.4	51.4	66.7
Cook, Ill.	57.9	33.8	26.9
DuPage, Ill.	55.5	17.9	20.0
Kane, Ill.	60.8	33.3	50.0
Lake, Ill.	60.7	47.4	75.0
McHenry, Ill.	54.1	25.0	33.3
Will, Ill.	61.7	18.2	0.0
Winnebago, Ill.	59.5	25.0	0.0
Johnson, Kan.	53.2	41.7	75.0
Wyandotte, Kan.	61.2	58.3	0.0
Clay, Mo.	59.6	75.0	—
Jackson, Mo.	55.5	28.9	11.1
Platte, Mo.	59.6	0.0	—
Bronx, N.Y.	73.3	55.8	60.0
Erie, N.Y.	52.2	23.5	33.3
Kings, N.Y.	58.9	46.7	50.0
Monroe, N.Y.	61.1	20.0	—
Nassau, N.Y.	43.2	29.7	48.5
New York, N.Y.	64.6	43.3	51.2
Onondaga, N.Y.	55.7	22.2	25.0
Queens, N.Y.	51.5	48.2	63.6
Richmond, N.Y.	66.2	30.0	40.0
Suffolk, N.Y.	52.2	41.7	54.5
Westchester, N.Y.	40.2	21.7	20.0
Multnomah, Ore.	60.4	22.0	54.5
Dallas, Tex.	50.9	21.4	0.0
Harris, Tex.	55.5	10.3	0.0
King, Wash.	61.1	27.3	16.6
Pierce, Wash.	61.8	28.6	0.0
Skagit, Wash.	78.9	—	—

TABLE **3** *continued*

County	Overall	Medical Malpractice	Ob-Gyn
Snohomish, Wash.	59.6	25.0	0.0
Spokane, Wash.	68.0	75.0	—
Yakima, Wash.	63.0	50.0	0.0

in only two counties—Clay County, Missouri, and Spokane County, Washington—were the malpractice rates higher than the overall rates. Both of these counties, however, reported only four malpractice cases.

Plaintiffs tended to be more successful in obstetrics and gynecology jury cases than in malpractice cases generally—but not much more successful (36.8 percent versus 32.4 percent). Table 3 shows that, for the 40 counties with obstetrics and gynecology jury cases, the success rates ranged from 0 in 14 counties to 75 percent in 2 counties. Again, the range narrows in counties with more cases.

It is worth noting, given our earlier use of Texas data for illustrative purposes, that the plaintiff success rate in obstetrics and gynecology cases in Dallas County, Texas—as in Harris County—was zero. Although not a part of our study, we also checked the success rate for Tarrant County, Texas (which borders on Dallas County and includes the cities of Fort Worth and Arlington) and found that it, too, was zero for the 1981–1985 period.

When we compare plaintiff success rates in obstetrics and gynecology cases with those in all jury verdicts, we find that in the majority of counties with obstetrics and gynecology cases (34 of 40) the success rate for all jury verdicts was higher. When we compare obstetrics and gynecology success rates with overall medical malpractice success rates, we find that in 18 of the 40 counties the obstetrics and gynecology success rate was higher. In 11 of those 18 counties, however, there were fewer than 10 obstetrics and gynecology cases. Of the remaining 7 counties, only 1 (Los Angeles County) was outside New York.

Types of Obstetrics and Gynecology Cases

Figure 1a shows a breakdown of the 364 obstetrics and gynecology verdicts by type of case, and Figure 1b presents the breakdown for the 134 successful obstetrics and gynecology verdicts. Labor and delivery made up the largest proportion (just over one-third) of all obstetrics and gynecology verdicts. There was a drop to the next largest proportion, which was hysterectomy at 11.5 percent. The next four types—pregnancy, cancer, tubal ligation, and abortion—were all clustered within a

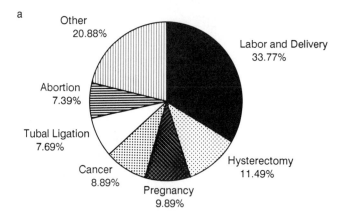

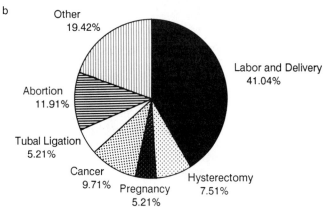

FIGURE 1.   a. Breakdown of ob-gyn cases by type ($N=364$). b. Breakdown of successful ob-gyn cases by type ($N=134$).

narrow range from about 7 to 10 percent. The remainder were scattered across a number of areas.

There is a slightly different pattern with respect to successful cases (Figure 1b). This pattern is important because it sets the parameters and provides the standards for negotiating the majority of disputes. Labor and delivery made up an even larger proportion of successful cases (41 percent) than of all verdicts (33.8 percent). There was, again, a large drop to the second largest proportion—in this instance abortion, which also made up a larger proportion of successful cases (11.9 percent) than of all cases (7.4 percent). Cancer was next, making up a slightly larger proportion of successful cases than of all cases (9.7 percent versus 8.9 percent). Fourth was hysterectomy, which made up a smaller proportion of successful cases than of all cases (7.5 percent versus 11.5 percent). Pregnancy and tubal ligation each accounted for 5.2 percent of the successful cases; for both, this is a smaller proportion than for all cases. Such contrasts indicate that there were important differences in plaintiff success rates for the respective types of obstetrics and gynecology cases; these differences will be discussed in detail later.

Severity of Injury

The severity of the patient's injury was assessed using the nine-point severity scale that has been used in a number of malpractice studies since the mid-1970s.[48] Table 4 presents a rough outline of the severity scale and some examples. The scale goes from no physical injury, to three categories of temporary injury, through four categories of permanent injury, to death. For ease of presentation, we collapsed these nine categories into four by keeping the two extremes—no physical injury and death—and collapsing all of the temporary injuries into one category and all of the permanent injuries into another (Figures 2a and 2b).

Nearly one-half of the obstetrics and gynecology cases involved a permanent injury, whereas only 8 percent involved no physical injury but, typically, some emotional injury. Generally, the injuries in obstetrics and gynecology cases were likely to be more rather than less severe. About 60 percent of the cases involved a permanent injury or death; 40.4 percent involved no physical injury or a temporary injury.

TABLE 4   Severity Scale

Severity of Injury	Examples
Temporary	
1. Emotional only	Fright, no physical damage
2. Insignificant	Lacerations, contusions, minor scars, rash; no delay in recovery
3. Minor	Infections, misset fracture, fall in hospital; recovery delayed
4. Major	Burns, surgical material left, drug side effect, brain damage; recovery delayed
Permanent	
5. Minor	Loss of fingers, loss or damage to organs; includes nondisabling injuries
6. Significant	Deafness, loss of limb, loss of eye, loss of one kidney or lung
7. Major	Paraplegia, blindness, loss of two limbs, brain damage
8. Grave	Quadraplegia, severe brain damage, lifelong care or fatal prognosis
9. Death	

SOURCE: National Association of Insurance Commissioners. 1980. Malpractice Claims: Final Compilation. Brookfield, Wis., p. 10.

a

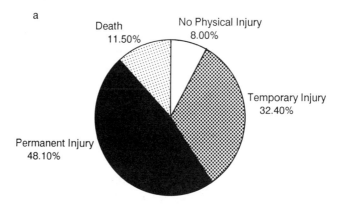

b

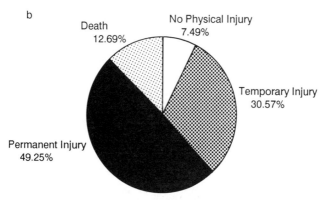

FIGURE 2. a. Breakdown of ob-gyn cases by severity of injury ($N=364$).
b. Breakdown of successful ob-gyn cases by severity of injury ($N=134$).

Juries were slightly more likely to decide in favor of the plaintiff in cases involving more severe injuries (Figure 2b). We can see this in the difference between the success rates (how often plaintiffs won) of more and less severe injuries in obstetrics and gynecology cases. Where the severity was death or permanent injury, the plaintiffs won at a rate of 38.2 percent, compared with 34.7 percent for no physical injury or temporary injury.

Cause of Injury

Figures 3a and 3b break down by cause of injury all obstetrics and gynecology verdicts and all successful obstetrics and gynecology verdicts. In collecting our data we used a set of categories that has appeared

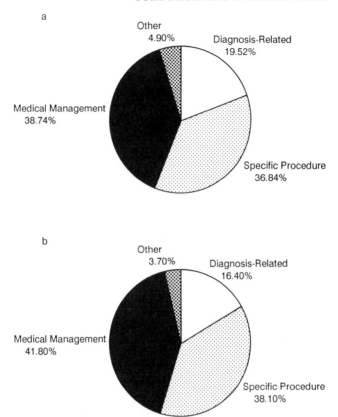

FIGURE 3. a. Breakdown of ob-gyn cases by cause of injury ($N = 364$). b. Breakdown of successful ob-gyn cases by cause of injury ($N = 134$).

repeatedly in the malpractice literature.[49] The most frequent cause of obstetrics and gynecology injuries was related to general medical management (the overall planning and handling of patient care, including cases involving the use and management of medications, failure in nursing management, and failure in physician planning and management). Injuries caused by a specific procedure or treatment (e.g., a surgical procedure) were a close second. Injuries caused by diagnostic problems (misdiagnosis or nondiagnosis) made up a much smaller proportion of the verdicts.

There was a roughly similar picture for successful obstetrics and gynecology cases (Figure 3b). Injuries related to medical management were again the largest percentage, but it was slightly higher than for all cases. Injuries caused by a specific procedure or treatment were again the second largest percentage, and that percentage was also slightly higher than for all obstetrics and gynecology cases. Diagnostic causes made up a smaller percentage of successful verdicts compared with all verdicts. Juries, it seems, were more likely to decide in favor of the plaintiff when the injury was caused by a specific procedure or was related to general medical management. The plaintiff success rates for these two categories were, respectively, 38.1 percent and 39.7 percent. The success rate for diagnostic problems was 31 percent.

Class of Injury

Another way of looking at the cause of injury is to break cases down by class of injury.[50] Injuries are divided into three classes. Class 1 injuries involve a new abnormal condition caused by the treatment or procedure, whether diagnostic or therapeutic (acts of commission). Figure 4a breaks down the 364 obstetrics and gynecology cases by class of injury, and it shows that 45.1 percent of the cases were class 1 injuries.

Another 29.7 percent of cases involved class 2 injuries, those resulting from incomplete diagnosis or treatment. Here, the original abnormal condition has not had the expected outcome because of acts of either commission or omission. Finally, 25.3 percent of the cases involved class 3 injuries, in which the patient suffers a new abnormal condition caused by incomplete prevention or protection (acts of omission).

The pattern changes somewhat for successful cases (Figure 4b). The proportion of class 1 injuries drops, as does the proportion of class 2 injuries. Class 3 injuries, on the other hand, increased, suggesting that juries were more likely to decide in favor of the plaintiff when the plaintiff suffered a new abnormal condition as a result of incomplete protection or prevention. This trend is evident in the plaintiff success rates. Class 1 cases had a success rate of 35.4 percent, class 2 cases a rate of 31.5 percent, and class 3 cases a rate of 45.7 percent.

Awards

Although the plaintiff success rates for obstetrics and gynecology cases were relatively low, awards tended to be high in those few instances in which plaintiffs were successful. The median award (expressed in 1985 dollars) was $390,000. To put this in perspective, the median award for all jury verdicts (not just medical malpractice) was less than $25,000 in one-half of the 46 counties studied.[51] Most personal injury cases, however, are not as severe as medical malpractice cases generally or obstetrics and gynecology cases specifically. The 25th award percentile for obstetrics and gynecology cases was $85,550; the 75th percentile was $1,665,000.

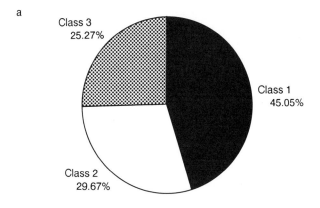

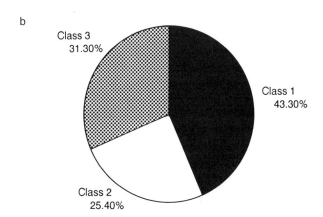

FIGURE **4.**   a. Breakdown of ob-gyn cases by class of injury (*N* = 364). b. Breakdown of successful ob-gyn cases by class of injury (*N* = 134).

A More Detailed View of the Shadow

In describing the general contours of the shadow cast by obstetrics and gynecology jury verdicts, we can see some interesting patterns emerge. Plaintiffs were not likely to win obstetrics and gynecology cases, but when they did win they were likely to be awarded large amounts of money by the jury. Most of the injuries brought before juries were alleged to have been caused by a specific procedure or by general medical management. The largest proportion of injuries involved the adverse effects of treatment—that is, acts of commission rather than omission. Finally, the verdicts were not equally distributed across the different types of obstetrics and gynecology cases. Disaggregating the obstetrics and gynecology verdicts by type of case and then examining cause, class, and severity of injuries together with success rates and awards for each type of case provide the means to explore the shadow's shape in more detail.

Table 5 presents data on number of verdicts; plaintiff success rate; cause, class, and severity of injury; and awards for the seven types of obstetrics and gynecology cases. It is the basis for our discussion of the shadow's details. For each type of case, Table 5 shows the number of verdicts and the plaintiff success rate, and presents two columns of data for each.

The left-hand column shows the percentage of all cases of a given type that fall into a particular category of injury. For instance, 50 percent of pregnancy cases were caused by a diagnosis-related injury. The number in parentheses just below (18) is the raw number of cases falling into the diagnosis-related category. The 50 percent figure is obtained by dividing the number of diagnosis-related pregnancy cases (18) by the total number of pregnancy cases (36). The total number for each type of case is given at the top of the column, just underneath the column heading.

The right-hand column shows the plaintiff success rate (the proportion of cases in which the jury awarded the plaintiff at least $1) for each category of injury. The success rate for pregnancy cases caused by a diagnostic problem was 11.1 percent. The number in parentheses just below (2) is the number of successful cases for that category. The 11.1 percent figure is obtained by dividing the number of successful cases (2) by the total number of cases in the category (18).

Pregnancy

Pregnancy-related cases made up 9.9 percent of the obstetrics and gynecology verdicts and had the lowest plaintiff success rate, 19.4 percent. Together with the low success rate, this type also presents a relatively modest award structure. The median award for pregnancy cases was $139,168, much less than the overall median of $390,000. The largest proportion of pregnancy cases (50 percent) had diagnosis-related causes of injury (e.g., failure to detect that a woman was pregnant or failure to suggest a pregnancy test when proposing a potentially teratogenic treatment for another problem), but the success rate for these cases was quite low (11.1 percent). Plaintiffs were most likely to be successful in cases involving medical management issues, for which the rate was 33.3 percent. Most pregnancy cases involved class 2 injuries (incomplete diagnosis or treatment), and plaintiffs were most successful in these cases. The severity of injury grouping was fairly evenly split between the combined categories of no physical injury and temporary injury, on the one hand, and permanent injury or death, on the other. Plaintiffs were more successful when the injury was more severe. The success rate for no physical injury and temporary injury combined was only 11.8 percent, while that for permanent injury or death was 26.3 percent.

Labor and Delivery

Labor and delivery cases made up the largest proportion (33.8 percent) of obstetrics and gynecology verdicts and showed one of the highest success rates and award structures. The plaintiff success rate for labor and delivery cases was 44.7 percent, compared with 36.8 percent for all obstetrics and gynecology cases. The median award was $1,665,000, far above the median of $390,000 for all obstetrics and gynecology cases and the median for any other type of obstetrics and gynecology case. In fact the labor and delivery median is higher than the 75th percentile for any other type of obstetrics and gynecology case and equal to the 75th percentile overall.

Nearly two-thirds of labor and delivery injuries were caused by problems in medical management (e.g., failure to adequately supervise or properly monitor). The success rate for these cases (47.5 percent) was higher than the rates for injuries with other causes—for example, the 35.7 percent for injuries resulting from a specific procedure (e.g., the improper use of forceps), the other major category of labor and delivery cases. One-half of the labor and delivery cases involved class 3 injuries (e.g., lack of monitoring); the plaintiff success rate in these instances was quite high, at 54.8 percent. The success rates for classes 1 and 2, in contrast, were 37.8 percent and 25.0 percent, respectively. Labor and delivery cases were more likely than overall obstetrics and gynecology cases to involve severe injuries: 78.9 percent of the cases involved permanent injury or death, and plaintiffs were successful in 46.4 percent of these cases. In comparison, 59.6 percent of total obstetrics and gynecology cases involved permanent injury or death, with a plaintiff success rate of 38.2 percent.

Abortion

Although abortion cases had the highest plaintiff success rate—59.3 percent—they had only a moderate award structure. The median award was $153,400, well below the overall median of $390,000; abortion cases

TABLE 5 Breakdown of Obstetrics and Gynecology (Ob-Gyn) Cases by Type According to Cause, Class, and Severity of Injury and Awards Made

Category	Pregnancy N=36, SR[a]=19.4 % (N)	SR (N)	Labor Delivery N=123, SR=44.7 % (N)	SR (N)	Abortion N=27, SR=59.3 % (N)	SR (N)	Hysterectomy N=42, SR=23.8 % (N)	SR (N)	Tubal Ligation N=28, SR=25.0 % (N)	SR (N)	Cancer N=32, SR=40.6 % (N)	SR (N)	Other Gyn N=76, SR=34.2 % (N)	SR (N)	Totals N=364, SR=36.8 % (N)	SR (N)
							Cause of Injury									
Diagnosis related	50.0 (18)	11.1 (2)	8.9 (11)	45.5 (5)	— (0)	—	4.8 (2)	0 (0)	3.6 (1)	0 (0)	84.4 (27)	44.4 (12)	15.8 (12)	25.0 (3)	19.5 (71)	31.0 (22)
Specific procedure	5.6 (2)	0 (0)	22.8 (28)	35.7 (10)	85.2 (23)	60.9 (14)	57.1 (24)	20.8 (5)	78.6 (22)	22.7 (5)	3.1 (1)	100.0 (1)	44.7 (34)	47.1 (16)	36.8 (134)	38.1 (51)
Medical management	41.7 (15)	33.3 (5)	65.0 (80)	47.5 (38)	14.8 (4)	50.0 (2)	28.6 (12)	33.3 (4)	14.3 (4)	50.0 (2)	12.5 (4)	0 (0)	28.9 (22)	22.7 (5)	38.7 (141)	39.7 (56)
Other	2.8 (1)	0 (0)	3.3 (4)	50.0 (2)	— (0)	—	9.5 (4)	25.0 (1)	3.6 (1)	0 (0)	— (0)	—	10.5 (8)	25.0 (2)	4.9 (18)	27.8 (5)
							Class of Injury									
Adverse effects (class 1)	16.7 (6)	16.7 (1)	36.6 (45)	37.8 (17)	48.1 (13)	53.8 (7)	76.2 (32)	25.0 (8)	50.0 (14)	14.3 (2)	9.4 (3)	66.7 (2)	67.1 (51)	41.2 (21)	45.1 (164)	35.4 (58)

Incomplete treatment (class 2)	61.1 (22)	27.3 (6)	13.0 (16)	25.0 (4)	40.7 (11)	63.6 (7)	11.9 (5)	40.0 (2)	21.4 (6)	33.3 (2)	90.6 (29)	37.9 (11)	25.0 (19)	10.5 (2)	29.7 (108)	31.5 (34)
Incomplete prevention (class 3)	22.2 (8)	0 (0)	50.4 (62)	54.8 (34)	13.0 (3)	66.7 (2)	11.9 (5)	0 (0)	28.6 (8)	37.5 (3)	— (0)	— (—)	7.9 (6)	50.0 (3)	25.3 (92)	45.7 (42)

Severity of Injury

No physical injury	25.0 (9)	11.1 (1)	4.9 (6)	16.7 (1)	22.2 (6)	66.7 (4)	— (0)	— (—)	10.7 (3)	33.3 (1)	— (0)	— (—)	6.6 (5)	60.0 (3)	8.0 (29)	34.5 (10)
Temporary injury	22.2 (8)	12.5 (1)	16.3 (20)	45.0 (9)	55.6 (15)	60.0 (9)	52.4 (22)	27.3 (6)	67.9 (19)	26.3 (5)	6.3 (2)	0 (0)	42.1 (32)	34.4 (11)	32.4 (118)	34.7 (41)
Permanent injury	44.4 (16)	25.0 (4)	62.6 (77)	44.2 (34)	18.5 (5)	60.0 (3)	42.9 (18)	16.7 (3)	17.9 (5)	20.0 (1)	65.6 (21)	34.4 (11)	43.4 (33)	30.3 (10)	48.1 (175)	37.7 (66)
Death	8.3 (3)	33.3 (1)	16.3 (20)	55.0 (11)	3.7 (1)	0 (0)	4.8 (2)	50.0 (1)	3.6 (1)	0 (0)	28.1 (9)	22.2 (2)	7.9 (6)	33.3 (2)	11.5 (42)	40.5 (17)

Awards (1985 dollars)

25th Percentile	$ 17,416	$ 189,000	$ 41,600	$ 27,750	$ 7,770	$ 254,782	$ 74,256	$ 85,550
Median	139,168	1,665,000	153,400	118,000	37,800	590,000	216,000	390,000
75th Percentile	832,000	3,330,000	390,000	500,000	93,000	1,107,000	864,998	1,665,000

*a*SR = plaintiff success rate.

also had the next-to-lowest 75th percentile, $390,000, far below the overall 75th percentile of $1,665,000. Nearly all of the abortion cases involved an injury tied to a specific procedure or treatment (negligence in the performance of the abortion itself), and plaintiffs were quite successful in specific procedure cases, with a success rate of 60.9 percent.

The greatest proportion of abortion cases (48.1 percent) involved class 1 injuries (a new abnormal condition such as a perforated uterus), and these cases had a success rate of 53.8 percent. The injuries involved in abortion cases tended to be less severe than those in obstetrics and gynecology cases overall. Of all obstetrics and gynecology cases, 40.4 percent involved no physical injury or temporary injury, with plaintiffs winning in 34.7 percent of of the cases. Of the abortion cases, in contrast, 77.8 percent involved no physical injury or temporary injury, with a plaintiff success rate of 61.9 percent in these combined categories. Plaintiffs were successful in just half of the six abortion cases in which the injury was a permanent one or death.

Hysterectomy

Hysterectomy cases had the second lowest plaintiff success rate, at 23.8 percent, and the second lowest award structure, with a median of $118,000. The largest proportion of the hysterectomy injuries (57.1 percent) was caused by a specific procedure (typically the surgical procedure itself), but plaintiffs were rarely successful in procedure cases—the success rate was only 20.8 percent. Most of the hysterectomy cases (76.2 percent) involved class 1 injuries (the adverse effects of medical intervention), but plaintiffs were successful in only 25.0 percent of these cases. The severity of injury for hysterectomy cases tended to be lower than that for obstetrics and gynecology cases overall: 52.4 percent of the hysterectomy cases involved temporary injuries (none involved no physical injury), compared with 40.4 percent overall in the two categories combined. Of those hysterectomy cases involving temporary injuries, plaintiffs were successful in only 27.3 percent. Plaintiffs were even less successful (20.0 percent) in cases in which the injury was permanent or in which death occurred.

Tubal Ligation

Tubal ligation cases had one of the lower plaintiff success rates, at 25 percent, and the lowest award structure. The 25th percentile was only $7,770, and the median was by far the lowest—$37,800, about one-tenth the overall median. Most of the tubal ligation cases (78.6 percent) involved injuries caused by a specific procedure (typically the surgical procedure itself), but plaintiffs were not often successful (22.7 percent) in these cases. One-half of the tubal ligation cases involved class 1 injuries (the adverse effects of medical intervention), and plaintiffs were rarely successful in these cases (14.3 percent). Tubal ligation cases involved the least severe injuries of all types of obstetrics and gynecology cases—78.6 percent involved no physical injury or temporary injury. Of these cases, plaintiffs were successful in 27.3 percent. Plaintiffs were even less successful (16.7 percent) in the tubal ligation cases involving permanent injury or death.

Cancer

Cancer cases had one of the highest plaintiff success rates (40.6 percent) and the second highest award structure, with a median of $590,000. The 75th percentile for cancer was $1,107,000, and the 25th percentile was $253,782. This 25th percentile for cancer cases was higher than any other and higher than the medians for all types of cases except labor and delivery.

Nearly all of the cancer cases (84.4 percent) had as their cause a diagnosis-related injury (e.g., failure to diagnose cervical cancer), and plaintiffs were successful in 44.4 percent of the diagnosis-related cases. An even larger proportion of cancer cases (90.6 percent) involved class 2 injuries (incomplete treatment or diagnosis); plaintiffs were successful in 37.9 percent of these. The cancer cases had the highest proportion of severe injuries; 93.7 percent involved permanent injury or death, and plaintiffs were successful in 43.3 percent of these cases. In contrast, no plaintiff was successful in the less severe cases.

Interpreting the Shape of the Shadow

Looking at the different types of obstetrics and gynecology cases in detail reveals important patterns in the shape of the shadow cast from the top of the dispute resolution pyramid. These patterns suggest that juries may not be as capricious in their handling of malpractice cases as some commentators have claimed. In fact if jury decisions were capricious, we should find little or no shape to the shadow—and certainly no identifiable patterns in the details. We might expect, on the one hand, similarity across types of cases—that juries make no distinctions; hence, all types of obstetrics and gynecology cases are handled the same. On the other hand, we might expect randomness when the different types of cases are compared—that is, no identifiable patterns. It is randomness that the rhetoric of malpractice says we should find.

The discussion of the data in Table 5 for the different types of obstetrics and gynecology cases indicates that neither randomness nor a general similarity was the rule. There were identifiable and important patterns in Table 5, and they became evident when comparisons were made among the different types of cases. Perhaps the most obvious place to start limning the details of the shadow's shape is with labor and delivery and cancer, the two groups with the highest award structures.

There were important similarities between the two types of cases. Along with high award structures, the two had relatively high plaintiff success rates (labor and delivery at 44.7 percent and cancer at 40.6 percent). For each, the greatest proportion of cases involved the more severe injuries (both had a percentage of cases involving permanent injury or death in excess of 78 percent). No other type of obstetrics and gynecology case had a percentage involving permanent injury or death that was as high as 54 percent. It would seem, then, that juries were more likely to decide in favor of plaintiffs and award more money in situations in which the injuries were more severe. The low success rates and low award structures for more severe injuries in hysterectomy and tubal ligation cases suggest that juries are not simply making emotional decisions based solely on severity of injury.

There were differences between labor and delivery and cancer cases in cause and class of injury as well, as one would expect. The predominant cause of injury for labor and delivery was medical mismanagement, and plaintiffs had a relatively high success rate for these cases (47.5 percent). Of the 55 successful cases, 69.1 percent involved medical management. The message from jury verdicts for physicians seems clear: greater care and diligence are needed in handling labor and delivery. For cancer cases, the predominant cause of injury involved diagnosis, and plaintiffs were quite successful (44.4 percent). Of the 13 successful cancer cases, 12 were diagnosis cases. Again, the message from jury verdicts seems clear. The predominant class of injury for labor and delivery was class 3—incomplete prevention or protection—and these cases made up 61.8 percent of the successful labor and delivery cases. For cancer cases, class 2 was predominant—incomplete treatment or diagnosis; these cases made up 84.6 percent of the successful cancer cases.

At the other extreme were the hysterectomy and tubal ligation cases, which had the lowest award structures and low plaintiff success rates, even when the injuries were more severe. For each type of case, the predominant cause of injury was a specific procedure, and plaintiffs were rarely successful in these cases (the hysterectomy success rate was 20.8 percent, the tubal ligation rate, 22.7 percent). For each type of case, class 1 injuries (a new abnormal condition as a result of medical intervention) predominated (hysterectomy at 76.2 percent and tubal ligation at 50 percent), and plaintiff success rates were low (25 percent and 14.3 percent, respectively). Perhaps most important, the injuries involved were not as severe as in labor and delivery or cancer. In both hysterectomy and tubal ligation cases, more than half the injuries were temporary or not physical. In both labor and delivery and cancer the percentage of these types of injuries was below 25 percent.

Juries, it seems, have not been awarding large amounts of money to plaintiffs in cases involving specific procedures and less severe injuries, nor have they been deciding cases overwhelmingly in favor of plaintiffs, even when injuries are more severe. The exception with regard to success rates was the abortion cases, which had a very high plaintiff success rate (59.3 percent), along with a high percentage of cases with no physical injury or temporary injury (77.8 percent). This pattern may have occurred because abortion is seen as a routine health care matter rather than a complicated procedure. Perhaps the reason for the difference in success rates for abortion cases as compared with hysterectomy cases and tubal ligation cases was in the jury's response to medical error in a situation in which the procedure involved is well known, relatively simple, and routinely used. Nonetheless, the award structure for abortion cases was modest.

These findings suggest that it is not the new technologies on the frontiers of medicine that were behind high awards or high plaintiff success rates but problems involving older, established technologies. Rather than reaction to the risks of the new, we may be seeing instead a lack of tolerance for mistakes in the use of the old and well established, especially in cases in which the injuries are more severe. This pattern becomes evident when we look more closely at the labor and delivery cases and at the subset of cases within this category that had the highest plaintiff success rate and the highest award structure. These were the cases involving the use of oxytocin, a drug used to induce labor. If improperly used, oxytocin can have serious, lifelong effects on the baby, such as paralysis, brain damage, and mental retardation.

Of the 123 labor and delivery cases, 28 included injuries caused by medications. Twenty-three of these involved the use of oxytocin; one involved the use of Demerol; one involved the use of "pain killers" otherwise unidentified; and the remaining three involved general allegations of overmedication.[52] To place the 23 oxytocin cases in proper perspective, some background on oxytocin is needed. The use of oxytocin to induce labor began in Germany in 1910 with the use of a pituitary extract. Parke-Davis began marketing oxytocin in this country in 1928 under the brand name Pitocin; Pitocin has traditionally been the brand of choice. In the 1950s a synthetic version was developed and was marketed by Parke-Davis under the same name.

Contraindications for the use of oxytocin began appearing regularly in the *Physician's Desk Reference* (PDR) in 1962[53] and by 1963 in the frequent Parke-Davis advertisements for Pitocin that appeared in the *American Journal of Obstetrics and Gynecology.*[54] The list of precautions grew throughout the 1960s and 1970s; by the 1970s they had begun appearing prominently in medical texts.[55] In 1978 the Food and Drug Administration (FDA) required that a warning notice be placed in or on the box in which the medication was packaged.[56] In January 1979 the FDA required that Parke-Davis submit a revised new drug application for Pitocin. The application was approved in November 1980. During the 1980s successive volumes of the PDR showed a lengthening and detailed list of precautions for the use of oxytocin. The dangers of oxytocin, then, were widely disseminated during the 1960s and 1970s, although they had been known for some time and were well documented in the medical literature by the early 1920s.[57]

Against this background we examined the 23 oxytocin cases in detail, comparing the allegations made about misuse of the drug with the list of precautions found in the PDR, in the Parke-Davis advertisements, and in other sources for the year in which the injury occurred. Sixteen of the 23 oxytocin cases alleged that the drug was used in a situation in which contemporary medical sources (PDR, manufacturer advertisements, and medical texts), as well as other sources,[58] said that it was contraindicated. Of these 16 cases, 6 involved inadequate supervision while using oxytocin, 4 involved fetal distress, 3 involved breech presentations, 2 involved pelvic disproportion, and 1 involved the taking of an inadequate patient history and the failure to do a blood test, either of which would have shown that the mother was diabetic.

Plaintiffs were successful in 14 of these 16 cases (plaintiffs were not successful in one of the breech cases and in one of the supervision cases). This compares with a success rate of 44.7 percent for labor and delivery cases generally and a rate of 36.8 percent for all obstetrics and gynecology cases. Of the 7 other oxytocin cases, those in which a contraindication was not evident in the case summaries, plaintiffs were successful in only 14.7 percent, lending credence to the juries' ability to distinguish a clear violation of the standard of care. The award structure for the 14 successful cases was very high. It ranged from $147,500 (in 1985 dollars) to $18,381,600. The median award was $3,660,000, compared with a median of $1,665,000 for all labor and delivery cases and a median of $390,000 for all obstetrics and gynecology cases.

Of the 16 cases involving contraindications, *all* resulted in permanent injury or death. When we examined them in more detail, using the full nine-point severity scale (see Table 4), we found that two cases involved a significant permanent injury and two involved death. The two cases in which plaintiffs were not successful involved grave permanent injury. In comparison, 78.9 percent of labor and delivery cases involved permanent injury or death, and 59.6 percent of all obstetrics and gynecology cases involved permanent injury or death. In the oxytocin cases then, juries appear to have responded in no uncertain terms to the misuse of an old, established technology whose limitations and contraindications were well known and widely disseminated.

CONCLUSIONS

The rhetoric of malpractice characterizes jury verdicts as irrational, unpredictable, uncertain, and decidedly pro-plaintiff in terms of who wins and the amounts of money awarded. As a consequence, radical changes in the civil justice system have been proposed and vigorously supported.

Our findings describe a very different shadow being cast by obstetrics and gynecology jury verdicts. Only a very small proportion of injury-causing medical errors ever leads to a claim against the physician, and fewer result in a jury trial. Of the small portion of obstetrics and gynecology errors that result in a jury trial, physicians win most of the time. When physicians lose, it is likely to be in situations that do not involve specific procedures but that do involve severe injuries and in situations involving older, well-established technologies. Awards, when plaintiffs are successful, may be high, but they are not excessive, given the seriousness of the injuries. The fact that it is older, established technologies rather than newer, frontier technologies that are generally involved suggests that targeted attempts at quality assurance may be more appropriate than radical tort reform in reducing obstetrics and gynecology malpractice litigation.

REFERENCES

1. Vander Kolk, K. 1985. Is that all there is? Am. J. Obstet. Gynecol. 152:139–144.
2. Ibid., p. 142.
3. Ibid., p. 140.
4. Ibid., p. 142.
5. Weir, B., J. Barlow, and B. Mydland. 1987. Hell in a bucket. Grateful Dead: In the Dark. AC-8452. New York: Arista Records.
6. Schulman, H. 1984. The doctor—Third parties. Am. J. Obstet. Gynecol. 149:624–627.
7. Johnson, S. 1985. Malpractice costs vs. health costs. New York Times. July 19, p. A-14.

8. American Medical Association, Council on Long-Range Planning and Development (with the cooperation of the American College of Obstetricians and Gynecologists). 1987. The future of obstetrics and gynecology. JAMA 258:3547–3553.

9. Vander Kolk. 1985, p. 140; see note 1.

10. Johnson, K. 1987. Beyond tort reform. JAMA 257:827–828.

11. Bowen, O. 1987. Congressional testimony on Senate Bill S. 1804. JAMA 257:816–819.

12. See, for example, K. Johnson. 1987; see note 10.

13. Ibid., p. 827.

14. Cohn, V. 1987. The price of malpractice: How the crisis harms the relationship between doctors and patients. Washington Post. March 12. Health Section, p. 10.

15. Bowen. 1987, p. 816; see note 11.

16. K. Johnson. 1987, p. 827; see note 10.

17. Ibid. See also American Medical Association—Specialty Society Medical Liability Project. 1988. A Proposed Alternative to the Civil Justice System for Resolving Medical Liability Disputes: A Fault-Based Administrative System. Chicago, pp. 7–8, 9, 81, 137–138, 140–142.

18. Burrow, D., and J. E. Collins. 1987. Insurance "crisis"—Texas style: The case for insurance reform. St. Mary's Law J. 18:759–796; Danzon, P. M. 1983. An economic analysis of the medical malpractice system. Behav. Sci. 1:39–55; Gifford, D., and D. Nye. 1987. Litigation trends in Florida: Saga of a growth state. Univ. Fla. Law Rev. 39:829–875.

19. Danzon, P. M. 1985. Medical Malpractice: Theory, Evidence, and Public Policy. Cambridge, Mass.: Harvard University Press.

20. General Accounting Office (GAO), U.S. Congress. 1986. Medical Malpractice: Case Study on Arkansas. GAO/HRD-87-215-1. Gaithersburg, Md. See also medical malpractice case studies on California, Florida, Indiana, New York, and North Carolina, also published in 1986; and see U.S. Department of Health and Human Services. 1987. Report of the Task Force on Medical Liability and Malpractice. Washington, D.C.: Government Printing Office.

21. See, for example, Galanter, M. 1986. Jury shadows: Reflections on the civil jury and the litigation explosion. Paper presented at the 1986 Warren Conference. Boston. June 12–15; Mnookin, R., and L. Kornhauser. 1979. Bargaining in the shadow of the law; The case of divorce. Yale Law J. 88:950–977.

22. Galanter, M. 1983. Reading the landscape of disputes: What we know and don't know (and think we know) about our allegedly contentious and litigious society. UCLA Law Rev. 31:4–71; Miller, R., and A. Sarat. 1980–1981. Grievances, claims, and disputes: Addressing the adversary culture. Law Soc. Rev. 15:525–566.

23. Brook, R., and R. Stevenson. 1970. Effectiveness of patient care in an emergency room. N. Eng. J. Med. 283:904.

24. Brook, R., M. Berg, and P. Schechter. 1973. Effectiveness of non-emergency care via an emergency room. Ann. Intern. Med. 78:333.

25. Danzon. 1985; see note 19.

26. California Medical Association and California Hospital Association. 1977. Medical Insurance Feasibility Study. San Francisco: Sutter.

27. Danzon. 1985, p. 20; see note 19.

28. National Center for Health Statistics. 1987. Summary: National Hospital Discharge Survey. Advance Data. Washington, D.C.: Government Printing Office.

29. Texas Almanac and Industrial Guide, 1986–1987. 1985. Dallas: The Dallas Morning News, p. 628.

30. Ibid.

31. California Medical Association and California Hospital Association. 1977; see note 26.

32. Danzon. 1985, p. 20; see note 19.

33. Ibid.

34. Ibid., p. 24.

35. Texas State Board of Medical Examiners. 1988. Medical Malpractice Statistics Reports. Austin.

36. Texas State Board of Medical Examiners. 1987. Medical Malpractice Statistics Reports. Austin.

37. May, M., and L. DeMarco. 1986. Patients and doctors disputing: Patients' complaints and what they do about them. Disputes Processing Res. Prog. Work. Pap. Ser. (University of Wisconsin Law School, Madison) 7(7):1.

38. National Association of Insurance Commissioners. 1980. Malpractice Claims: Final Compilation. Brookfield, Wis.

39. Texas State Board of Medical Examiners. 1988; see note 35.

40. American Hospital Association. 1985. Annual Survey Standard Report. Chicago.

41. Galanter. 1986, p. 19; see note 21.

42. Ibid., p. 2.

43. Galanter, M. 1981. Justice in many rooms. J. Legal Pluralism 19:1–47.

44. Daniels, S. 1986. Civil juries, jury verdict reporters, and the going rate. Paper presented at the annual meeting of the Law and Society Association. Chicago. May 29–June 1.

45. Daniels, S., and J. Martin. 1986. Jury verdicts and the "crisis" in civil justice: Some findings from an empirical study. Justice Sys. J. 11:321–348.

46. Daniels. 1986; see note 44.

47. Daniels and Martin. 1986; see note 45.

48. See, for example, California Medical Association and California Hospital Association. 1977; note 26. National Association of Insurance Commissioners, 1980; note 38. Danzon. 1985; note 19.

49. For example, California Medical Association and California Hospital Association. 1977; see note 26. Danzon. 1985; see note 19.

50. California Medical Association and California Hospital Association. 1977; see note 26. National Association of Insurance Commissioners. 1980; see note 38. Danzon. 1985; see note 19.

51. Daniels and Martin. 1986, p. 338; see note 45.

52. Rucker, M. P., and C. Haskell. 1921. The dangers of pituitary extract. JAMA 76:1390–1393.

53. Physician's Desk Reference. 1962, 1963, and 1985. Oradell, N.J.: Medical Economics.

54. Parke-Davis Pharmaceutical Co. 1963. [Advertisement]. Am. J. Obstet. Gynecol. 87:16.

55. Zackey, J. 1980. Pitocin: Lethal agent in obstetrical malpractice. Trial 16:57–59.

56. Food and Drug Administration, U.S. Department of Health and Human Services. 1978. FDA Drug Bulletin 1. Washington, D.C.: Government Printing Office.

57. Goodman, L., and A. Gilman. 1956. The Pharmacological Basis of Therapeutics. New York: Macmillan; Rucker and Haskell. 1921; see note 52. Woodbury, R. A., W. F. Hamilton, B. E. Abreu, R. Torpin, and P. H. Friedman. 1944. Effects of posterior pituitary extract, oxytocin (Pitocin) and ergonovine hydracrylate (Ergotrate) on uterine, arterial, venous and maternal effective placental arterial pressures in pregnant humans. J. Pharmacol. Exp. Ther. 80:256–263.

58. Ibid.

The Virginia Birth-Related Injury Compensation Act: Limited No-Fault Statutes as Solutions to the "Medical Malpractice Crisis"

JAMES A. HENDERSON, JR.

In this chapter I accept as a premise that we face a "medical malpractice crisis" and examine possible solutions. The crisis presumably consists of significant increases in the number and value of medical malpractice claims, the mounting unavailability to medical care providers of liability insurance, and the growing possibility that such providers will respond to these circumstances by cutting back on or refusing altogether to provide needed health care services. Although several possible solutions are considered, limited no-fault statutes such as the recently enacted Virginia Birth-Related Neurological Injury Compensation Act are the major focus of concern. Statutes of this sort aim at the hottest of the hot spots in the medical malpractice crisis, replacing traditional tort liability with narrowly defined no-fault compensation programs. Because such statutes focus on areas where the problems are the greatest, presumably they offer relief where it is most needed.

To assess the potential benefits of such approaches, I compare these limited no-fault approaches with traditional tort liability and with more comprehensive alternative compensation systems. The peculiar strengths and weaknesses of each system are identified, and comparisons are drawn between and among the various approaches. I conclude that, although no-fault alternatives to traditional tort are feasible in the medical malpractice area, limited no-fault statutes such as that of Virginia are of questionable social value. Even assuming that the medi-

194

cal malpractice crisis exists and demands legal change, such approaches may well create more problems than they solve.

SIGNIFICANT FEATURES OF TRADITIONAL TORT AND ALTERNATIVE COMPENSATION SYSTEMS

General Descriptions of the Systems

Traditional Tort Liability System

As masters of ceremonies are often disposed to say, the traditional tort system needs no introduction. In the medical malpractice area the basis for liability is negligence on the part of the health care provider. The plaintiff typically claims that the provider deviated in a dangerous way from the standards of the relevant branch of the medical profession, causing injury to the plaintiff.[1] The plaintiff brings his claim by filing a complaint in a court of law and by going to trial in cases that fail to be settled. A greater percentage of medical malpractice claims actually reach trial than is typical in other areas of tort liability,[2] perhaps reflecting the relatively higher costs to the defendants of appearing to admit fault by agreeing to a settlement.

Medical malpractice trials are lengthy and expensive. In cases brought to trial juries typically decide at the close of the evidence whether the health care provider was or was not negligent, with negligence being determined by reference to the standards of care currently adhered to by the medical profession.[3] A finding of liability requires the jury to assess the damages to be awarded to the plaintiff. Reflecting the relatively high expense of bringing these cases to trial, verdicts and judgments tend to be greater in malpractice claims than in tort claims generally.[4] Many claimants receive little or nothing from this process; those who succeed, however, tend to recover substantial judgments.

Comprehensive No-Fault Alternative

In contrast to the traditional tort liability system a comprehensive no-fault alternative to compensating the victims of medically related accidents would define ahead of time the adverse medical outcomes for which compensation would be awarded and would process claims in an administrative rather than a judicial setting.

A useful example of such a system, which I will use in this analysis for comparison, is the Designated Compensable Event (DCE) project of the American Bar Association (ABA). In 1977 the ABA Commission on

Medical Professional Responsibility recommended that its innovative alternative subcommittee explore the possibility of implementing an enterprise liability system based on a predefined list of adverse outcomes arising from medical treatment.[5] The DCE system proposed in 1979 at the end of that study rests on the assumption that for most medical treatments and procedures it is possible to identify those adverse outcomes over which medical professionals exert significant control—that is, adverse outcomes that are usually although not invariably avoidable under good quality medical care.[6] Prepared ahead of time by medical researchers and reviewed by teams of clinicians, the list of adverse outcomes, or designated compensable events, forms the basis of an enterprise liability system in which patients suffering one or more of the listed outcomes are paid out of the proceeds of insurance, which are attained ahead of time by the relevant providers, without having to show that the providers were at fault. For outcomes on the DCE list, the enterprise liability remedy would be exclusive. For outcomes not listed, patients would have access to the traditional tort system.[7]

Presumably, such a DCE compensation system would be broad in its coverage and would be implemented either by contract (e.g., a contract between a health maintenance organization and its subscribers) or by statute (imposed on all providers of medical care in the relevant jurisdiction). To date, the DCE program has not been implemented in any jurisdiction.

Limited No-Fault Statutes

In contrast to the DCE approach limited no-fault statutes such as the Virginia Birth-Related Neurological Injury Compensation Act focus narrowly on a specifically defined set of injuries—in the case of the Virginia statute, on injuries to the brain or spinal cord of infants caused by the deprivation of oxygen or by mechanical injury occurring in the process of birth.[8] The Virginia statute imposes its terms on the patients of physicians and hospitals opting ahead of time to participate in the program. For covered claims, the statute excludes any and all rights to recover in tort. Claims are processed administratively, and recoveries are limited by preestablished schedules. The fund from which compensation payments are made is maintained by annual public assessments on participating physicians, hospitals, and physicians generally, with nonparticipating physicians paying at a reduced but not insubstantial rate. Liability insurers are also assessed, based on the extent of their involvement in writing certain kinds of insurance in the state. The Virginia statute took effect on January 1, 1988. It is not yet clear how, in fact, it will operate.

How Is Each System Implemented? What Is the Source of Each System's Legal Authority?

The Traditional Tort System

The traditional system of medical malpractice tort claims rests in the common law, modified here and there by statute. A few states in recent years have modified the common-law tort system somewhat radically,[9] but the traditional common-law tort system survives as the underlying basis of medical malpractice liability in all American jurisdictions. In most states the common-law tort system governing medical malpractice claims has survived statutory tinkering largely if not completely intact.[10]

The DCE System

The DCE system proposed by the ABA study might be implemented by statute, but it need not be. Indeed, the ABA study assumed that a DCE pilot program would be adopted initially and experimentally by contract, probably by a health maintenance organization, which would include such a compensation system in its basic contract with subscribers. It is more difficult to envision individual health care providers and their patients adopting this contractual system, given the inclination of American courts to review such provider-patient contracts with suspicion after the fact of injury.[11]

If a large health maintenance organization were to decide to implement a DCE approach, it might be well advised to seek legislation authorizing but not necessarily imposing such contracts and purporting to "guarantee" the validity of contracts that conform to statutorily established guidelines. In the alternative a state legislature, confronting what it deemed to be a serious malpractice crisis, might enact legislation imposing the DCE approach on health care providers and patients generally. Given the unavoidably controversial nature of such a proposal, and the serious implications of its enactment, many advocates of the DCE approach understandably prefer that it be implemented initially through the contract mechanism.

The Virginia No-Fault Statute

The Virginia approach imposes its no-fault compensation scheme on everyone in the commonwealth, in the sense that physicians or hospitals who choose to participate in the program thereby impose that scheme on their patients unilaterally.[12] The Virginia statute does not require participating physicians or hospitals to notify patients ahead of time that the statute has replaced any and all rights they might otherwise have under the tort system in the event of a birth-related neurological injury.

What Triggers Liability? What Events Are Compensable?

The Traditional Tort System

In a medical malpractice action brought under traditional tort principles the plaintiff must show that the health care provider failed to conform to the commonly accepted standards of his or her particular branch of the medical profession.[13] That is, the plaintiff must show provider fault. The standard is relatively vague, and most often the question of liability is for the jury to decide on general instructions. Given the relative vagueness of the standards of care to be applied,[14] the tribunal "stick builds" a description of the compensable event in each case and then applies that standard to the facts. Relatively little is decided ahead of time; trials in court provide the context in which the law and fact are developed.

The DCE System

In contrast to the traditional tort system, the DCE system prepares a comprehensive list of adverse outcomes ahead of time, describing in detail those outcomes that will warrant compensation for injuries suffered. Various criteria are used in specifying outcomes to be included on the list: for example, outcomes must be generally although not invariably within the control of health care providers. The DCE system should provide incentives, through the differential pricing of insurance premiums, to providers to exercise care in controlling the number and extent of adverse outcomes. The more frequently any given provider experiences such outcomes, the higher his or her liability premiums will be.

The key to success under the DCE approach is the specificity with which the outcomes are described. Most of the value judgments must be made ahead of time, leaving substantially mechanical judgments of fact to be determined case by case. For example, the DCE system might describe a particular type of plaintiff (excluding the very young, the very old, and patients who are particularly at risk of adverse outcomes) and a particular type of health care service (an appendectomy or a tonsillectomy) and then describe the adverse outcome as "death during the operation or during the period of immediate recovery." The phrase "the period of immediate recovery" must be described specifically in terms of time and space.[15] Once this event is included on a list of designated compensable events, death from any source—even death resulting from collapse of the operation room ceiling—would generate a valid claim for compensation. The system must avoid addressing questions of proximate cause under vague standards; most claims must be handled routinely and administratively if significant reductions in the costs of processing claims are to be achieved.[16]

Controllability by the health care provider is not the only criterion. One might include on the list of designated compensable events adverse outcomes that are not generally within the control of providers but that result from medical procedures that are close substitutes for procedures whose outcomes are included. Unless such substitutable procedures are included, providers will have incentives to substitute procedures that do not lead to DCE claims for compensation in place of procedures that do, thus skewing the system.[17] It should be noted that the ABA commission contemplated in its report a DCE system that would cover a wide range of medical procedures. Because the DCE list is intended to provide such coverage, it must be concerned with substitution effects.

The Virginia No-Fault Statute

The Virginia statute defines the statutory phrase "birth-related neurological injury" as follows:

"Birth-related neurological injury" means injury to the brain or spinal cord of an infant caused by the deprivation of oxygen or mechanical injury occurring in the course of labor, delivery or resuscitation in the immediate post-delivery period in a hospital which renders the infant permanently nonambulatory, aphasic, incontinent, and in need of assistance in all phases of daily living. This definition shall apply to live births only.[18]

Several observations regarding this statutory language are in order. At first blush, the language seems sufficiently specific to avoid controversy when applied case by case; one may wonder, however, whether the phrase "caused by the deprivation of oxygen or mechanical injury" raises difficult questions of causation. Can physicians determine relatively easily and unambiguously when brain or spinal cord injury has and has not been caused by such deprivation or injury? If not, then the seeming specificity of the statute may dissolve in a morass of administrative haggling.[19]

Apart from this question concerning causation, the description of the compensable events in the Virginia statute seems very narrow in scope when compared with the longer, more comprehensive list of compensable events in the proposed DCE system. The Virginia statute appears to have addressed the hottest issue in the malpractice crisis in that jurisdiction, aiming narrowly at a type of injury that one may reasonably assume leads to significant liability under the traditional tort system. Reacting to the narrowness, one begins to wonder why this particular outcome was picked to receive such unusual treatment. Even if the compensable outcome in the Virginia statute can be determined fairly simply, thereby reducing transaction costs, questions of fundamental fairness remain. The DCE system arguably would provide greater benefits in the aggregate to persons injured in the course of receiving medical treatment than are provided by the traditional tort system. To be sure, the DCE system would pay badly injured claimants less than the traditional tort system would pay successful tort plaintiffs in similar cases, but the number of victims receiving compensation under the DCE system would, presumably, be greater than the number under traditional tort. Indeed, one of the arguments favoring the DCE system is that it can provide more benefits in the aggregate, given the significant reductions in the costs of processing the claims. Those costs, many of which are legal costs, can be transferred back to victims in the form of larger aggregate compensation.

In contrast the Virginia statute will almost certainly result in a net reduction in aggregate recoveries. If one is reasonable in assuming that severe birth-related neurological injuries were chosen precisely because they are among the most troublesome and costly to the providers of obstetric health care, one can be confident that the aggregate compensation paid out to those who suffer such injuries will be less than the aggregate compensation (including compensation to the lawyers involved, in the form of attorneys' fees) paid out under the traditional tort system. Thus, the Virginia statute appears to be primarily a "reduce the liability costs of providers" approach, rather than a "reduce the transaction costs of handling medical malpractice claims" approach. The manner in which the Virginia statute describes the compensable event raises questions regarding the objectives being served by this narrowly focused compensation scheme. I shall address the question of goals and objectives in a later discussion, but problems begin to appear almost at the outset.

Who Pays? Who Gets Paid?

The Traditional Tort System

Under traditional tort, the provider found at fault, or the provider's liability insurer, pays the tort claims. The victim of the malpractice, or the victim's family, receives the payments. Providers are presumably free to carry or not to carry liability insurance. The problem of liability insurance being unavailable to providers has surfaced from time to time and has prompted a variety of institutional responses.[20]

The DCE System

Under the DCE approach, compensation insurance would be mandatory for providers participating in the system. Presumably, such insurance might be subject to deductibles that would cause the providers to carry some part of the insurance load themselves. The claimants or their survivors would receive the compensation.

The Virginia No-Fault Statute

The Virginia statute calls for payments out of a specially established, state-maintained fund.[21] The patients or their survivors receive the benefits.[22]

How Is the System Funded?

The Traditional Tort System

Under traditional tort, health care providers presumably obtain liability insurance to cover most if not all of their exposure to liability. For those providers who do not carry insurance or whose insurance does not cover all of their exposure, the providers satisfy liability judgments from their own resources. For victims of adverse outcomes who cannot establish provider fault, the losses fall on the victims themselves or on their families, to be covered to a limited extent by loss insurance and more generally by personal and community resources.

The DCE System

Under the DCE system, compensation insurance is mandatory for participating health care providers. In addition the DCE approach determines the insurance premiums on the basis of the provider's experience rating, helping to establish incentives for providers to exercise care.[23] For adverse outcomes not included on the DCE list, victims and their families are left to the traditional tort system, with its combination of liability insurance or self-insurance for the providers and loss insurance or self-insurance for the victims, families, and communities involved.

The Virginia No-Fault Statute

An interesting feature of the Virginia scheme is the creation of a fund from which compensation payments to successful claimants are made.[24] All physicians in Virginia are taxed annually at a rate sufficient to provide a portion of the fund necessary to make compensation payments; participating physicians, hospitals, and liability insurers pay at relatively higher rates.[25] It is puzzling why nonparticipating physicians must pay to subsidize the providers who actually participate in and benefit directly from the Virginia no-fault system.

How Are the Benefits Measured?

The Traditional Tort System

Under traditional tort, the amount that a successful plaintiff recovers is tailored to fit the facts of each particular case. Out-of-pocket expenses are allowed, including medical expenses and lost earnings.[26] In addition, losses of future earning potential are allowed,[27] as are awards for intangible elements of loss such as conscious pain and suffering.[28] An important feature of the traditional tort system is the collateral source rule, which refuses to deduct amounts received by the plaintiff from outside sources when calculating the tort damage award.[29] Outside sources may, by contract, arrange ahead of time with their insured to be repaid out of the tort recovery, but the tort system ignores such collateral in calculating tort damages. The plaintiff's attorney traditionally is paid out of the damage award. These contingent fee agreements reduce the net amounts going to successful plaintiffs, but they ensure a ready source of remuneration with which to recruit some of the best trial lawyers to bring tort actions.

A distinctive feature of traditional tort is that damage awards are paid in a lump sum; that is, they are paid all at once, when judgments in favor of successful plaintiffs are satisfied. Statutory movement toward payments over time (periodic payments) has occurred in recent years,[30] but most often, lump-sum payments are made.

The DCE System

Instead of tailoring awards to the facts of each case, the DCE system schedules awards. The schedules are geared to the facts of the individual case only in the sense that amounts vary with the severity and duration of the claimant's injury. Recovery for pain and suffering is either eliminated altogether or severely limited. Compensation awards under the

DCE system have an off-the-rack quality, compared with damages awards under traditional tort.

Consistent with most alternatives to traditional tort, the DCE system might well consider eliminating the traditional collateral source rule;[31] that is, the DCE compensation system could be secondary to other sources of compensation. This need not be the case, however. In theory, the DCE system might be considered the primary source of compensation, with other sources seeking reimbursement from DCE awards for amounts paid to successful claimants. The latter approach would enhance the providers' incentives to exercise care in controlling adverse outcomes. Abolishing the collateral source rule subsidizes the DCE compensation system, blunting the incentive to take care.

Regarding the questions of how the awards are paid (in a lump sum or over time) and how the plaintiff's attorneys are paid, the DCE system could take a flexible approach. It probably makes sense to favor periodic payouts of compensation awards because these may better help injured plaintiffs cope with their financial setbacks.[32] Such payouts, when imposed unilaterally, however, are vulnerable to attack as being overly paternalistic. If claimants prefer to receive their benefits in a lump sum, perhaps they should be entitled to do so. Attorneys' fees might be handled as they are under traditional tort, coming from the compensation awards, with sterner oversight by the agency that would administer the compensation system.

The Virginia No-Fault Statute

Under the new Virginia statute, compensation awards are scheduled.[33] Compared with the proposed DCE system, however, they appear to be aimed as much at reducing the aggregate cost of compensation as they are at reducing administrative overhead. Thus, a successful claimant will receive, for loss of earnings from the age of 18 to the age of 65, an amount equal to half the average weekly wage in the Commonwealth of Virginia for workers in the private, nonfarm sector.[34] As with many if not most no-fault systems, the Virginia system eliminates the collateral source rule, at least for out-of-pocket expenses.[35] The statute provides for the award of reasonable attorneys' fees.[36]

By What Processes of Decision Are Claims Handled?

The Traditional Tort System

The two major processes for resolving most tort claims are settlement and adjudication. Settlement occurs in the context of bargaining between plaintiffs and defendants in individual cases. Most tort claims that are not settled are tried before juries of laypersons who decide the major factual disputes and apply the relevant law. Expert testimony plays a significant role in medical malpractice cases. Given their heavy reliance on expert testimony, medical malpractice cases are relatively expensive to adjudicate.[37] The costs to the defendants, both in time taken to testify at the trial and mental and emotional upset, are substantial.[38]

More than half of the states have introduced procedural reforms that require specially established screening panels to hear medical malpractice claims before plaintiffs take the claims to court.[39] The effects of screening panels vary from jurisdiction to jurisdiction. In many states, the recommendation of the screening panel is admissible at a later trial. Presumably, when the administrative screening panel concludes that the claim is groundless, it hurts the plaintiff's chances if and when the claim is taken to court. Faced with such a disincentive, some plaintiffs may be persuaded to carry their claims no further.

The DCE System

As with most alternatives to traditional tort, the DCE system relies on nonadjudicative administrative procedures to handle claims. Given the very specific guidelines regarding which claims are and which are not compensable, these administrative bodies would presumably exercise little discretion and juries would not be required. The greatest savings of time and scarce resources should occur here. Compared with trials requiring many weeks and many thousands of dollars to accomplish, administrative hearings would take less time and consume fewer resources. When claimants are unhappy with the outcomes reached in the administrative process, judicial review is available.

The Virginia No-Fault Statute

Under the Virginia statute, as with the DCE proposal, an administrative agency processes and handles compensation claims. In the Virginia scheme, the Industrial Commission hears the claims and makes the primary dispositions.[40] Both the Board of Medicine and the Department of Health evaluate claims initially and report their reactions to the commission;[41] a special medical advisory panel reviews each claim and reports its recommendations at least 10 days prior to the hearing before the commission.[42] The commission itself (or the single member thereof assigned to hear the claim) determines the validity of each claim, subject to subsequent review by the full commission and ultimate judicial review in the Court of Appeals.[43]

How Exclusive Is the Remedy Provided? What Is the Interface with Other Compensation Systems?

The Traditional Tort System

Traditional tort may be fairly characterized as being unconcerned with whether other liability or compensation systems exist. Tort law simply moves forward with its own agenda and lets the chips (in terms of other possible sources of compensation for accident victims) fall where they may. This attitude is reflected clearly in the collateral source rule.[44] These observations regarding the self-centeredness of traditional tort should not strike the reader as startling. After all, traditional tort was, at least apart from contract and until the advent of workers' compensation, the only "game" in town.[45] Thus, the problem of managing the interface between and among liability and compensation systems is a significant problem that systems other than common-law tort must face.

The DCE System

Like all alternatives to common-law tort, the DCE system must be concerned with how its remedies react with potential remedies in tort. To avoid horrendous problems of adverse selection—problems that arise when plaintiffs may, after the fact of injury, pick and choose which compensation system offers the best deal—the DCE remedy must be exclusive and replace the tort remedy once the adverse outcome has occurred. I have explored elsewhere the practical problems of how the DCE system should attempt to work with the tort system.[46] For example, when a tort claim is brought prior to the bringing of a DCE claim, what effect on the tort claim should the possibility of a DCE claim have? Should a claimant be allowed to bring both a DCE claim and a tort action simultaneously? Clearly, these problems must be worked out. One way or another, however, the DCE claim when available must be the primary and exclusive claim.

Thus far, I have considered only ex post (after the fact of injury) elections regarding which system to pursue. What about ex ante (before the fact of injury) decisions regarding whether to opt into the DCE system? Should potential victims of adverse medical outcomes (patients) have an opportunity, prior to the delivery of the relevant medical care services, to elect to be covered by the DCE system? If the DCE system were implemented by contract, some degree of ex ante election would be available, perhaps in the form of health maintenance organization subscribers opting, as a group, to participate. At the least, patients should be told ahead of time that they are bound by the terms of an applicable

DCE system. In any event it is important for drafters to understand that the problem of the interface between compensation and tort must be addressed not only ex post but also ex ante.

The Virginia No-Fault Statute

Regarding ex post elections of coverage by victims of birth-related neurological injury, the Virginia statute makes the compensation remedy exclusive of all other rights and remedies of the affected infant and his or her representatives.[47] The way the statute is worded, it appears that, if a claim were to be brought in tort for injuries presumably covered by the statute, that claim would be barred by an appropriate motion before the court, pending resolution of the compensation claim under the statute. The statute of limitations on the tort claim is tolled (barred from running) pending the resolution of the no-fault claim.[48] If the no-fault claim is allowed, that is the end of the matter. If the claim is denied, presumably a tort action might follow. The one exception to the exclusivity of the no-fault remedy relates to the plaintiff's right to bring a tort action notwithstanding coverage under the statute when he or she can show, on clear and convincing evidence, that the covered physician or hospital intentionally or willfully caused the birth-related neurological injury.[49] Even such a claim of intentional fraud will be barred if it is brought after an award under the compensation statute becomes conclusive and binding.[50]

Interestingly, the Virginia statute does not address the process by which the families of victims are notified, ex ante, regarding whether their rights to recover for injuries will be limited to the compensation scheme. The statute describes the process by which physicians and hospitals opt into the program, but there is no explicit mention of how the families of potential victims—patients of such participating physicians and hospitals—learn of the fact that their physician or their hospital has opted to be covered. This may be a serious flaw in the Virginia plan as originally enacted, and the legislature should give it due attention.

COMPARING AND CRITIQUING THE GOALS AND OBJECTIVES OF THE THREE LIABILITY-COMPENSATION SYSTEMS

The Traditional Tort System

The major goals of tort law appear to be deterrence of wastefully risky conduct and compensation of accident victims injured by overly risky behavior. These assertions are admittedly couched in instrumental terms; they view tort law as a means that serves ends outside itself. Some writers have objected to this instrumental perspective and have insisted that tort law serves noninstrumental, essentially fairness values.[51] Rather than rehearse the arguments on each side, this discussion adopts a primarily instrumental perspective. I believe that the compensation objective is overplayed in much discussion of the objectives of tort. Tort law never has taken as its primary goal the compensation of accident victims. Far too many constraints on liability are imposed for that to have been the overriding goal. Rather, by defining tortious conduct in limited ways, tort law appears primarily to be aimed at creating incentives for actors to invest adequately in care. From that perspective, traditional medical malpractice tort law aims at helping to keep doctors on the right track—at pressuring them to conform to the standards of their profession. Toward that end, negligence is defined in terms of the general concept of "standards of the medical profession," and each case is then resolved on its own particular facts. Juries play a significant role, not only in determining what happened but also in determining the appropriate standard.[52]

In theory, the tort system creates just the right incentives for care. Over time, the adjudicative process generates patterns of outcomes that help to pressure physicians to optimize the social welfare. In practice, the vagueness of the standards and the slippage built into the jury system cause the traditional tort system to impose liability to some extent on a random rather than a systematic basis. Health care providers know in a general way that carelessness and negligence will expose them to liability, but the tort system does not enable them to know with any certainty where lines will be drawn later on. The system thus takes on some of the characteristics of a lottery. To the extent that this process occurs, tort law may further goals of deterrence, but it does so only haphazardly and at high transaction costs. It would not be patently absurd to conclude that the major (if not the only) beneficiaries of traditional tort are trial lawyers.

The DCE System

In contrast to traditional tort, the DCE system aims more at compensating the victims of adverse medical outcomes. It maintains a commitment to deterrence by defining compensable events in terms of adverse outcomes that health care providers may control through the exercise of care. Thus, the DCE approach compensates victims only when to do so would, over time, raise the levels of care among health care providers. The DCE system, unlike the traditional tort system, is concerned—one might say primarily concerned—with the reduction of transaction costs. Its administration through agencies other than courts helps to reduce transaction costs. The specificity with which adverse outcomes are described ahead of time reduces the time and resources consumed in applying the standards to any particular case. Benefits are spread more evenly among victims, though not so evenly as they would be spread under universal loss insurance. Most important, by adopting the designated compensable event approach, the system reduces the intangible "sting and upset" costs to health care providers, costs that the traditional tort system generates. The DCE approach awards compensation not because the provider has been at fault but because a previously designated adverse outcome has occurred.

Admittedly, the DCE system provides off-the-rack justice, compared with the traditional tort system. The boundaries drawn by the DCE list are bright; cases falling on either side of the boundaries may be treated very differently, even though, when viewed from a traditional perspective, they are quite similar. Yet the costs of arbitrariness are presumably more than offset by the reductions in other kinds of costs, including transaction costs and "provider upset" costs. Admittedly, a DCE system would require periodic updating of the list as new medical procedures become available. The traditional tort system, in contrast, automatically adjusts for such developments insofar as standards applicable in any given case are developed at trial. Once again, the trade-off is between reductions in transaction costs and tailoring remedies to fit individual cases. In theory, the tort system might be preferable, inasmuch as it ensures that, in every instance, the "punishment fits the crime." Given the slippage and the open-endedness of the tort system, however, it is doubtful that traditional tort in fact lives up to its billing. The DCE system would substitute a somewhat more rough-and-ready system that delivers greater aggregate benefits for a tort system that delivers less case-by-case substantive justice than is often assumed.

The Virginia No-Fault Statute

When one turns to the Virginia statute to assess its goals and objectives, the narrowness of the defined compensable event creates suspicion that the major objectives were not deterrence and compensation but rather the riddance of an especially troublesome (from the physician's perspective) subset of malpractice claims. One imagines a growing concern, reflected in the news media, that physicians offering birth-related care will refuse to do so if their exposure to traditional tort liability continues. Alarmed, the Virginia legislature reacts by enacting statutory relief for that very narrowly defined constituency. Presumably, the measure will reduce significantly the aggregate amounts paid in premiums by obstetricians and related specialists. Interestingly, all other categories of physicians in Virginia are required to contribute annually to subsidize their colleagues in the field of obstetrics.

At the conference at which this chapter was presented orally, a physician observed in open discussion that determining the cause of any neurological injury at the time of birth would be impossible for any dedicated finder of fact. Perhaps the statute assumes that the medically oriented panels that will decide the issue of causation in these cases will know it when they see it. It will be recalled that the DCE outcomes were drafted to eliminate, wherever possible, reliance on such notions of causation—for example, death *from any cause whatever* during elective surgery would bring compensation, even if the roof of the operating room fell in on the patient.[53] In contrast, the Virginia statute limits the compensable adverse outcome to injuries caused by certain rather narrowly defined sources.

Admittedly, to include all newborn infants who suffer severe neurological injury would be to include many who were doomed to that fate regardless of the care provided during birth. It might also be more difficult in this context than in the DCE system's elective surgery context to weed out high-risk patients ahead of time when defining who among the larger group may recover for adverse outcomes from the medical procedure. But the Virginia statute's reliance on causation will probably cause considerable mischief.

Viewed from the perspective of one seeking to discern its overall goals and objectives, the Virginia statute strikes this observer as something of an odd duck. Surely the medical malpractice crisis in Virginia has larger dimensions than birth-related neurological injury. Will the next subset of physicians that manages to capture the ear of the Virginia legislature receive a similarly beneficial "solution"? Over time, will that state be peppered with these focused legislative responses to crises, reflecting those subsets of the medical profession that have substantial political clout? From a tort scholar's perspective, talking about the overall goals and objectives of the Virginia statute presents analytical difficulties at best.

CONCLUSION

Based on the foregoing comparative analysis, and assuming once again that we face something of a crisis under the traditional tort approach to medical malpractice, a DCE system or one like it would be preferable to the more limited, focused approach of the Virginia compensation statute. Simply stated, the Virginia approach may reflect too much politics and too little concern for the appropriate goals and objectives of liability and compensation systems. Indeed, I would not be surprised if Virginia courts were to question the constitutionality (under the state constitution) of such a narrowly focused statute. Beyond the question of constitutionality, the act is problematic in several regards, all of which have been touched on earlier: its reliance on the element of causation may present intractable problems of proof; its disregard for patients' need to know about their rights ahead of time is troubling; the manner in which the scheme is funded, with its major beneficiaries being subsidized generally by physicians in Virginia, raises questions; and the overall impression that the act is aimed primarily at reducing obstetricians' exposure in the hottest of medical malpractice hot spots gives me reason to wonder if this statute may not be the first of a series of similar legislative responses to vocal, politically influential constituencies.

One test that any reform proposal should be prepared to pass is whether reasonable patients would agree to it before receiving care. Arguably, they would agree to a broad-based DCE system that delivered more to them in the aggregate than does the existing tort system. In contrast, I rather doubt that patients would agree ahead of time to being bound by the Virginia scheme. If my hunch is correct, then one may question the fundamental soundness of this hot-spot approach to solving the malpractice crisis. Ordinarily, I have little patience with the proclivity of state courts to set aside legitimate attempts by state legislatures to solve otherwise insoluble impasses in our traditional tort system. The Virginia statute tests my patience in quite the opposite direction.

REFERENCES AND NOTES

1. McCoid, A. H. 1959. The care required of medical practitioners. Vanderbilt Law Rev. 12:549–632.
2. Danzon, P. 1985. Medical Malpractice: Theory, Evidence, and Public Policy. Cambridge, Mass.: Harvard University Press, p. 56; Danzon, P. 1982. The Frequency and Severity of Medical Malpractice Claims. Santa Monica, Calif.: Rand Corp.
3. Pearson, R. N. 1976. The role of custom in medical malpractice cases. Ind. Law J. 51:528–557.
4. Danzon. 1985, pp. 53–55; see note 2.
5. Report of the American Bar Association Commission on Medical Professional Liability. 1977. Chicago: American Bar Association.
6. For a description of the DCE approach, see Henderson, J. A., Jr. 1982. The boundary problems of enterprise liability. Md. Law Rev. 41:659–694. The concept of general avoidability is closely akin to the premise underlying the common law tort doctrine of res ipsa loquitur, which permits an inference of negligence based on the fact of the injury itself. See, generally, Kaye, K. 1979. Probability theory meets res ipsa loquitur.

Mich. Law Rev. 77:1456–1484. As used in the DCE context, the avoidability concept would be broadened somewhat to include all instances in which the rate of adverse outcomes differs significantly between good and bad medical care, regardless of whether bad care was responsible for a large majority of adverse outcomes. The basis for this more liberal approach to the controllability concept is the DCE system's formal abandonment of the fault principle—all that really matters is that strict liability imposes significantly different liability costs on good and bad medical care providers on a long-term basis, regardless of the absolute likelihood in specific cases that either class of providers was negligent.

7. Barring plaintiffs' access to the traditional tort system for unlisted outcomes was felt to be unjustifiably harsh and thus politically unacceptable. Given the overlap between the DCE lists and the sorts of injuries for which recovery could be had under traditional negligence principles, the DCE system would presumably eliminate a substantial portion of the existing medical malpractice caseload; if the transaction costs associated with the cases based on unlisted outcomes were deemed unacceptable, the DCE statute might increase the plaintiff's burden of proof to, for example, clear and convincing evidence.

8. Va. Code Ann. §§ 38.2-5000 to 38.2-5021 (Supp. 1988). Hereafter, sections of the statute will be referred to by section number.

9. See, for example, Conn. Gen. Stat. Ann. §§ 52-225a to 52-225d, 52-251a, 52-251e, 52-557m to 52-557n, 52-568, 52-572h (West Supp. 1988). See, generally, Manzer, N. L. 1988. Note, 1986 tort reform legislation. Cornell Law Rev. 73:628–652.

10. For a brief summary of the most commonly encountered statutory modifications, see Danzon. 1985, p. 35; note 2. See also Grad, F. P. 1986. Medical malpractice and the crisis of insurance availability: The waning options. Case Western Reserve Law Rev. 36:1058–1098, esp. pp. 1076–1085.

11. Henderson, J. A., Jr. 1986. Agreements changing the forum for resolving malpractice claims. Law Contemp. Prob. 49:243–251.

12. § 38.2-5002.

13. McCoid. 1959; see note 1. Pearson. 1976; see note 3. See also the accompanying text.

14. In theory, at least, adoption by the courts of the medical profession's standards ought to render the legal standard more specific than merely "reasonableness under the circumstances." See, generally, Henderson, J. A., Jr. 1976. Expanding the negligence concept: Retreat from the rule of law. Ind. Law J. 51:467–527. Compared with the even brighter lines typically drawn by no-fault systems, the medical malpractice standard leaves room for considerable slippage.

15. For example, the period might include time spent in the postoperative recovery facility in the hospital, terminating when the patient leaves that facility.

16. Henderson. 1982, pp. 670–673; see note 6. These costs also include the costs to providers, in the form of mental upset and reputational damage, of being accused of incompetency.

17. The assumption here is that exposure to tort liability is in either instance remote.

18. § 38.2-5001.

19. To avoid the haggling, administrators of the Virginia scheme might routinely deny coverage or recognize coverage only when they sense that the underlying malpractice tort claim is strong. In either event, such a pattern of reactions would defeat the purported objectives of the statute.

20. Danzon. 1985, pp. 107–112; see note 2.

21. §§ 38.2-5015 to 38.2-5021.

22. Section 38.2-5001 of the act defines "claimant" to include the injured infant, his or her legal representative, or the estate of a deceased infant.

23. "Experience rating" means that each insured's premiums reflect the insured's claims experience; the more claims an insured has experienced in the past, and thus the more claims he or she is likely to experience during the period covered by the insurance, the higher his or her liability insurance premiums will be.
24. §§ 38.2-5015 to 38.2-5021 and accompanying text.
25. §§ 38.2-5019 to 38.2-5020.
26. Henderson, J. A., Jr., and R. Pearson. 1988. The Torts Process. Boston: Little, Brown, pp. 202–204.
27. See, for example, *Holton* v. *Gibson,* 402 Pa. 37, 166 A.2d 4 (1960).
28. See, for example, *Walters* v. *Hitchcock,* 232 Kan. 31, 697 P.2d 847 (1985).
29. Danzon. 1985, pp. 166–170; see note 2. For a recent critique of the collateral source rule in the context of medical malpractice claims, see, generally, McDowell, B. 1985. The collateral source rule—The American Medical Association and tort reform. Washburn Law J. 24:205–226.
30. Danzon. 1985, pp. 163–166; see note 2.
31. See Danzon. 1985; note 2. McDowell. 1985; see note 29.
32. Danzon. 1985, pp. 164–165; see note 2.
33. § 38.2-5009.
34. § 38.2-5009(3).
35. § 38.2-5009(1)(a) to (d).
36. § 38.2-5009(4).
37. Danzon. 1985, pp. 186–207; see note 2.
38. See note 16 and accompanying text. See also Bell, P. A. 1984. Legislative intrusion into the common law of medical malpractice: Thoughts about the deterrent effect of tort liability. Syracuse Law Rev. 35:939–993, esp. pp. 985–992.
39. Henderson. 1986, pp. 249–250; see note 11.
40. § 38.2-5008.
41. §§ 38.2-5004(B) to 38.2-5004(C).
42. § 38.2-5008(B).
43. §§ 38.2-5010 to 38.2-5011.
44. See Danzon. 1985; note 2. McDowell. 1985; see note 29. See also accompanying text.
45. The exception in the text for contract-based liability claims is, of course, a significant one. The interface between tort and contract remains interesting to this day. See, for example, the chapter by Richard Epstein in this volume.
46. Henderson. 1982, pp. 685–689; see note 6.
47. § 38.2-5002.
48. § 38.2-5005.
49. § 38.2-5002(C).
50. Ibid.
51. See, for example, Fletcher, G. P. 1972. Fairness and utility in tort theory. Harvard Law Rev. 85:537–573.
52. For example, expert witnesses often disagree regarding what procedures are called for by "good medical care."
53. See text following note 15.

Legislative Proposals on Medical Professional Liability Regarding the Delivery of Maternal and Child Health Care

W. HENSON MOORE

The cost of medical malpractice litigation, settlements, insurance, and defensive medicine has become a major factor in the rapidly rising cost of health care, jeopardizing affordable high-quality medical care. This phenomenon also has its social costs. The present tort system is a litigation lottery system—some malpractice victims win big, while most get nothing. Unfortunately, medical malpractice is a very complex issue without coordination or consensus among interest groups as to either its causes or possible solutions. Most agree, however, that it is a major problem.

Almost all state legislatures have responded to this near-crisis situation by changing their professional liability statutes.[1] In some states these measures have had no quantifiable effect, whereas in others they have slowed the escalation rate of the problem but have not solved it. The frequency and size of the claims have continued to rise in spite of the states' efforts. The federal government, by way of both the legislative and the executive branches, has also attempted to find solutions to the medical malpractice dilemma. Although many bills have been introduced, Congress so far has not seriously considered a major medical malpractice reform measure, nor does it appear ready to do so in the near future. The U.S. Department of Health and Human Services has also suggested solutions.

Provider organizations have not been as inactive. The American Medical Association (AMA) and the American Hospital Association (AHA), for example, recently issued their own proposals. Several other interested private organizations have issued reports analyzing the problem and offering possible solutions. In my opinion, none of these proposals offers a definitive, cost-efficient, and equitable solution. An examination of each proposed solution reveals serious flaws. Most of the solutions aim solely at reform of the tort system; they do not address its basic problems or its unfairness to patients and providers. Litigation simply is not the most humane or efficient way to compensate victims of malpractice.

• Persons advocating a private contract approach to medical care ignore the basic relationship between physicians and patients. Physicians and patients are not equally situated parties dealing with the same amount of information, which would allow them to arrive at a mutually acceptable bargain. Patients often either cannot or do not want to understand the risks they face. Illness, especially when it entails surgery, produces great stress and emotion in the patient. A contract-based system therefore will not solve the current malpractice problem.

A no-fault system, advocated by others, is simply financially infeasible now, given the uncertain state of medical advancement.[2] A no-fault scheme would require paying compensation for a large number of events that are not now actionable and that are most likely unavoidable. Physicians and health care providers may be held liable on the basis of a standard of which they had no knowledge. Rather than the no-fault or contract proposal, some reasoned, equitable approach is desperately needed.

THE PROBLEM

To help Congress address the public policy issues involved in the medical malpractice crisis, the U.S. General Accounting Office (GAO) analyzed national medical malpractice claims data.[3] The GAO estimated that 73,472 medical malpractice claims were closed in 1984. Approximately 43 percent of them terminated in an indemnity payment, the total of which for the year was $2.6 billion. In addition to indemnity payments, insurers incurred about $807 million in costs to investigate and defend claims; 57 percent of these costs went for claims that were closed without an idemnity payment.[4]

In obstetrical cases, however, indemnity payments were made for almost half the claims that involved injuries occurring at birth, and the claimants received the highest average payments of any class of claims. Although only 10 percent of all paid claims were for obstetrical errors, those claims accounted for 27 percent of the total payments. Of the obstetrical claims, 7.5 percent were for medical malpractice, and about 24 percent of those were for failure to identify fetal distress. About 9 percent of all the patients in the analysis were injured at birth, and 62 percent of those experienced obstetrics-related errors. Although obstetrician-gynecologists were named in 12 percent of all malpractice claims, insurers paid only 46 percent of these claims.[5]

Only about 8 percent of the indemnity payments involved a structured payment, alone or in combination with a lump sum payment, which totaled $951.4 million. The expected yield of these payments is estimated at $3.8 million. Payment of claims usually took more than one year; the more severe and costly cases took longer to resolve. Of the claims involving one provider, about 88 percent were settled before trial, and about 38 percent of those were settled after the claim was filed but before suit was instituted.[6]

The average payment increased with the severity of the injury. At the same time, the variance in awards and settlements was greater for more severe injuries. Patients sustaining injuries for which an economic loss could be estimated recovered an amount equal to or more than that loss in 70 percent of the claims. Patients with economic losses in excess of $100,000, however, recovered, on average, less than their actual loss. In about half such claims for which plaintiff attorneys' fees could be estimated, fees ranged from 30 to 40 percent of the expected value of the indemnity; in about 96 percent of the claims, the fee represented 40 percent or less of the indemnity payment.[7]

These facts indicate an inefficient and expensive situation at best.

STATE REFORMS

During the mid-1970s, the increasing cost and lack of availability of medical malpractice insurance prompted 49 states to enact various reforms. As part of a case study into the effects of various state reforms, the GAO asked organizations representing physicians, hospitals, insurers, and lawyers in six selected states how they perceived the malpractice insurance problem. For comparison, the GAO obtained countrywide claims data from the St. Paul Fire and Marine Insurance Company, the largest medical malpractice insurer in the United States.[8]

Most of the changes made by these six states were in response to the crisis of the mid-1970s and focus on tort reforms that were designed to ensure the availability and reduce the cost of malpractice insurance. Rather than enacting reforms to change the way public bodies and peer groups regulate health care providers, the states' responses change the way in which the insurance industry is regulated or help to develop realistic consumer expectations about the health care delivery system. Some states found that these reforms helped moderate upward trends in the cost of insurance and the average amount paid per claim, especially in cases in which the state had enacted a statutory cap on malpractice awards and a pretrial screening process. Other states found that the reforms had little effect. No state found that its reforms entirely solved the medical malpractice problem.[9]

Despite this moderating effect, insurance costs for physicians and hospitals increased dramatically after 1980, as did the number of malpractice claims filed and the average amounts paid. From 1980 to 1986, the cost of malpractice insurance often increased much more rapidly than the consumer price index and the medical care index. During this same period, medical malpractice insurance costs for obstetricians increased 345 percent in New York, 395 percent in Florida, and 547 percent in North Carolina. The frequency of claims reported against physicians and hospitals also increased. Between 1980 and 1984 rates for physicians and hospitals insured by St. Paul increased 56 percent and 71 percent, respectively, while the average paid claim against those physicians and hospitals increased by 102 percent and 137 percent, respectively. In the six states selected for the case study, the total number of claims increased in a range of 19 percent to 92 percent. Increases in the average claim paid on behalf of physicians ranged from 63 to 129 percent, and claims paid on behalf of hospitals increased from 33 to 141 percent. Insurers' costs to investigate and defend malpractice claims also increased in all six states.[10]

The years 1986 and 1987 brought another cascade of state legislation: 39 states enacted or strengthened medical malpractice reform laws. Again, these measures were directed mainly toward reform of the tort system. The one exception occurred in the Commonwealth of Virginia, which passed a novel piece of medical malpractice legislation, the Virginia Birth-Related Neurological Injury Compensation Act. This law takes birth-related neurological injuries out of the tort system and puts them into a program similar to workers' compensation, which assures lifetime care for infants with severe neurological injuries.[11]

This legislation was passed in response to the shortage of obstetrical services caused by the crisis in availability of malpractice insurance for obstetricians. To receive payment under the act, the infant must be profoundly injured, the treating physician must be a participating physician and must deliver obstetrical services at birth, the birth must occur in a participating hospital, and there must be a finding that malpractice occurred. A claim must be filed with the Virginia Industrial Commission, which holds a hearing at which only the claimant and the program are parties. Every claim is reviewed by a panel of uninvolved physicians, one of whom must be available to testify at the hearing.

If the claimant is successful at the hearing, the program will pay, directly to the infant, its lifetime medical, hospital, rehabilitative, and custodial expenses; its living expenses at a predetermined amount from age 18 years; and the reasonable expenses incurred in filing the claim, including discovery costs. Noneconomic damages are eliminated, punitive damages and the collateral source rule are abolished, and the statute of limitations on claims is markedly reduced.

There are several advantages to this no-fault system. First, physicians do not have a financial and professional threat to their practice. There is, however, automatic referral of all claims to the licensing agencies of the physicians and hospitals to ensure quality of care. If a review of the claim gives reason to believe the care provided was substandard, these agencies will investigate and take appropriate action. Because this is essentially a peer review process, it will be much more equitable for physicians.

Second, the system will attract private insurers, who earlier had fled Virginia in large numbers, back into the obstetrical malpractice insurance market. Third, it eliminates the uncertainty of the tort recovery system, providing a way to give lifetime care to infants who might otherwise have received nothing. The plan is financially feasible because it is predicted that only about 40 children per year will qualify.

This piece of legislation is the only one of its genre in existence today. It has taken a landmark first step toward a solution to the insurance crisis facing obstetricians—and it has done so not by tinkering with the tort system but by removing this particular injury from the tort system. At the same time, children and their families who are covered by this bill have the guarantee of swift and certain compensation. In some cases, years of judicial battling toward an uncertain result will be saved.

Although it is too early to determine the success of this legislation, it raises several questions. If the concept is sound, why was it limited to birth-related neurological injuries? Furthermore, will there be efforts to expand the program to cases with an undesirable result but no clear malpractice? Last, if it is expanded to undesirable results, would it then become a true no-fault system and would the cost become a problem as the universe of claims grows?

The various legislative measures passed by the states in 1986–1987 vary widely in terms and effect, but all make some degree of change in the tort system. Despite their variety, they can be grouped into a few general categories. Those measures aimed at tort reform include limitations on the doctrine of joint and several liability, limits on noneconomic damages, limits on punitive damages, modification of the collateral source rule, limits on attorneys' fees, imposition of screening panels, special statutes of limitations, structured payments of high verdicts, and restrictions on pie-in-the-sky "ad damnum" claims for damages.[12]

Of these reforms, four are most likely to have a positive effect on the cost of medical malpractice defense and the high cost of medical malpractice insurance. These are (1) modification of the collateral source rule, (2) abolition of joint and several liability, (3) limitations on attorneys' fees, and (4) limits on damages. It must be remembered, however, that adoption of any combination of these four measures in any one state will only slow the increase in defense and settlement costs rather than stop it. Malpractice litigation remains in the tort system.

Collateral Source Rule

This rule prohibits the introduction of evidence at trial that the plaintiff has been compensated for damages by anyone other than the defendant. The rule has been criticized as allowing plaintiffs to collect twice for the same injury. A 1982 Rand study found that relaxation of the collateral source rule reduced potential verdicts by 18 percent.[13]

Many states have abolished or modified the collateral source rule in medical malpractice actions.[14] Such measures may have only a modest effect on verdict amounts, however, because a reduction made to offset other damages received will not affect the higher cost noneconomic damage items. The effect on settlement negotiations, however, should be greater, as defense counsel can argue reductions in basic claims during this process.

Joint and Several Liability

Under the doctrine of joint and several liability, each defendant is liable for the full amount of the damage award, regardless of his or her degree of fault. During the last few years, many states have enacted laws limiting joint and several liability. Some states retain the doctrine only in cases in which the plaintiff is completely free of fault. This policy is unlikely to have a significant impact on medical malpractice claims because in the typical case the plaintiff is helpless in the face of a medical problem and must rely entirely on the health care provider's expertise. Thus, the opportunity to develop a convincing argument of contributory negligence simply is not present.

In states that have modified or abolished joint and several liability, medical malpractice claims may be more significantly affected. Medical care frequently involves an effort by a team of providers, that is, nurses, doctors, and other health care professionals. The plaintiff will no longer have the advantage of being able to lump together all of the provider defendants in the eyes of the jury, point to a tragic result, elicit expert testimony that the different mistakes by the various providers taken together caused the injury,[15] and then hope that liability will be assessed jointly and severally against all defendants, allowing a collection from the single, deep pocket.

Besides restricting the plaintiff's access to deep-pocket defendants, the amended statutes will affect the burden of proof. Usually, the quality and specificity of the expert testimony needed to make the causal proof that a series of acts or omissions by different defendants taken together caused injury are very low.[16] Under this reform, the plaintiff will have to prove that the component acts of *each* defendant had a specific causal relation to the injury. This requirement will force the court, as well as the jury, to focus on the issue of causation. The length of, complexity of, and margin of error in expert testimony will increase dramatically, opening up opportunities for legal and factual attack on the plaintiff's case. As these opportunities are discovered and utilized in the course of litigation, with the concomitant increase in expense and risk to the plaintiff of going to trial, the result should be a decrease in verdict and settlement amounts, as well as the possibility of fewer suits.

Limitations on Attorneys' Fees

Many states have enacted laws to limit compensation to counsel. A few states rely exclusively on court supervision to limit fees, but most adopt contingency fee schedules tied to the amount collected. These schedules vary widely in effect and amount. Usually, the percentage collected goes down as the damage award increases. Some states (e.g., Florida) further tie the fee schedule to the stage of the proceeding at which the money is collected.[17]

These limitations are intended to ensure that plaintiffs are not victimized and that attorneys do not receive more than a fair share of awards intended to redress injuries. Limitations on attorneys' fees will reduce defense costs two ways. First, with respect to minor injuries, in cases in which the size of an award is likely to be small, limits on fees can discourage unnecessary litigation, reducing the inclusion of peripheral defendants and the pursuit of marginal cases or marginal claims. Because most states allow from 33.3 to 40 percent on the first $50,000, however, it is unlikely that there will be a dramatic effect on the number of small damage claim suits.

Second, and more important, fee limits are likely to have a profound impact on the settlement process. As more of the money in a settlement reaches the plaintiff, total settlement amounts should decline. The Rand study observed that limits on contingent fee schedules cut the average settlement by 9 percent.[18] In large cases, the effect should be even more pronounced. For example, under a flat 40 percent contingency fee system, a plaintiff who is willing to settle for $600,000 must receive a $1 million settlement. Under the Massachusetts schedule, the same plaintiff would receive $600,000 with a $860,000 settlement, a decrease of 14 percent.[19] As the total settlement increases, this percentage savings will increase: a plaintiff who is willing to settle for $2 million must receive $3.3 million under a 40 percent contingency fee system as opposed to to $2.726 million under the Massachusetts schedule, a reduction of approximately 18 percent.[20]

Limits on Damages

Limits on damages fall into three categories: restrictions in pleadings, structured payments, and—the most controversial—caps on amounts. Many states have adopted one or more of these measures. The first prohibits pleading pie-in-the-sky ad damnum damage amounts in medical malpractice complaints. The Rand study found this cut the average settlement amount by 25 percent and raised the portion of cases dropped before verdict by 12 percent.[21]

Structured verdict payments allow large verdicts to be paid out over time, thus reducing the real cost of the verdict. The practice also allows the insurer to purchase an annuity rather than pay out a single large sum of money. Many states require, or authorize at the discretion of the court, structured payments for verdicts over a certain amount. Thus, there is an incentive to settle for a lower amount in cases in which the plaintiff has suffered serious future damages yet wants immediate access to a lump sum.[22]

Of the three types of damage reform measures, caps on damages have the greatest potential for reducing noneconomic losses.[23] The Rand study found that a cap on verdicts reduced the average projected settlement by 25 percent, raised the portion of cases dropped by 12 percent, and reduced the number of cases going to trial by 5 percent. In addition, the number of very high verdicts (over $1 million) decreased in states with such caps.[24]

The ability of such caps to withstand challenge under federal and state constitutions has been mixed. Six state courts have struck down such legislation: Idaho, Illinois, New Hampshire, North Dakota, Ohio, and Texas.[25] Only California and Indiana have upheld the constitutionality of such caps.[26] The U.S. Supreme Court has denied review in the California case.[27] The challenges have been based on federal and state rights to equal protection, substantive due process, access to courts, and trial by jury. Similar arguments have been made in challenges to caps on attorneys' fees.[28] As a general trend, in instances in which the jury is allowed to specify the portion of the award that relates to noneconomic damages, these limits are upheld.

ALTERNATIVES TO TORT REFORM PROPOSALS

Reforms aimed at modifying the present tort system ignore the problems inherent in it. One proposal for an alternative to the tort system was the Moore-Gephardt bill, introduced in the 98th and 99th Congresses as H.R. 5400 in April 1984 and as H.R. 3084 in July 1985, respectively. This bill suggested a speedy, low-cost, equitable process that could eliminate time-consuming expensive litigation and provide a rational recovery system that would take the injury out of the tort system. The bill was not a no-fault proposal, as providers were not required to make tenders for any and all maloccurrence. Rather, they would make offers when they recognized they were at fault or there was a plausible claim that was likely to be accepted by a jury. The proposal retained the central principle of tort law that compensation should be based on faulty behavior rather than provide compensation for all bad outcomes occurring in the course of providing health care.

The proposal introduced incentives for providers to pay compensation voluntarily to victims more quickly than the victims could recover through litigation and avoided requiring providers to pay for all adverse outcomes; however, it did not include a legislative delineation of the circumstances under which payment must be made. Rather, compensation was tied to each provider's assessment of responsibility. When a provider concluded that negligence might be found in court, the provider could make a commitment to pay compensation based on the injured patient's net economic loss, thereby foreclosing tort litigation. If the provider did not choose to pay, the patient retained his right to have the provider's liability determined under the current tort system, subject to full tort damages, including pain and suffering and other noneconomic costs. The desire to avoid the litigation lottery and its potentially very high payouts, not to mention the cost, distraction, and unpleasantness of litigation, was thought to motivate providers to make reasonable offers to settle on the basis of fairer, more controlled payments.

Under the proposal, the payment process would work as follows. A health care provider would have the option within 180 days of an adverse outcome (that is, one that could give rise to a malpractice action) to make a commitment to pay the patient's net economic loss resulting from the event. The patient would be entitled to complete reimbursement of out-of-pocket losses, such as lost wages and extra medical expenses, minus any payment available to the patient from third parties, such as the patient's health insurance. Counseling, treatment for pain, prostheses, rehabilitation, and other costs would be reimbursable. The compensation payments would be made periodically, as the patient's economic loss accrued, so it would not be necessary to know or estimate the amounts actually covered at the time the commitment is made.

Once the provider had made such a commitment, the patient's right to pursue a malpractice claim under the tort system would be terminated. Thus, in exchange for the provider's prompt assumption of responsibility for economic loss, the patient would lose his or her legal claim to non-economic loss. In the absence of a timely commitment the patient could either proceed with a malpractice action exactly as under current law or obtain speedy arbitration of the issue of the provider's fault and, if successful, recover net economic loss.

Providers would make such offers because they know the tort system does not work to their advantage. The opportunity to avoid the litigation lottery is limited to 180 days. Because the outcome itself starts the clock, the proposal encourages providers to develop measures for identifying possible malpractice quickly. Under the tort system, providers and their insurers receive no certain reward for prompt intervention and may be tempted to wait for the patient to make a claim, all the while hoping that the problem never comes to light. Under this proposal, providers and insurers could mitigate damages only by identifying and acknowledging any malpractice quickly, informing patients, and taking remedial measures.

In some instances, prompt provider action would be impossible: for instance, problem childbirth, erroneous diagnosis, and failure to provide informed consent may all take time to discover. In such cases, the provider's option to make a payment commitment would be triggered by the receipt of a claim rather than by the event itself.

The commitment to pay for the patient's net economic loss as it occurs would be fully enforceable as a matter of law. Net economic loss is a reasonable standard of compensation, prompt payment of which would greatly benefit injured patients. It would encompass the out-of-pocket cost of continued medical and hospital care, rehabilitation, nursing care, wage loss, housekeeping services, and adaptation of the patient's house and car, as well as reasonable attorney fees incurred in advising the patient. Furthermore, no question about the reasonableness of the promise could delay the commitment because the qualifying tender is not a fixed estimate of future damages but a commitment to pay specified elements of loss in full as they come due.

If one potential defendant made a commitment under the proposal, the patient would not retain the right to sue other potential defendants in the same alleged malpractice. Otherwise, the plaintiff would get the best of both worlds—prompt payment of out-of-pocket loss without litigation plus the ability to sue any or all of the other participants for duplicate damages. If anything, payment from one defendant would enhance the plaintiff's capacity to hold out against the others.

To avoid this result, the bill permits providers to join together in the commitment to pay the patient's net economic loss. Thus, if a hospital commits to pay a patient, it may designate a physician as a contendere. A physician tenderer, likewise, may designate the hospital. Either may also designate, for example, a drug or equipment manufacturer. Joining the potential defendants in the commitment makes it unnecessary for the patient to determine which defendants may be culpable. The victim is also protected from the mutual finger pointing that is so common (and expensive) among tort defendants. On the other hand, the victim cannot play one defendant off against another.

The joint participants could decide among themselves how they will share the obligation owed to the patient. Because these parties are likely to be represented by insurance companies that deal with one another on an ongoing basis, they will in most cases agree on their respective shares, based on private rules of thumb and practiced negotiation. If they could not agree, such disputes would go to arbitration to determine the parties' respective shares on the basis of relative negligence. This procedure not only could be conducted more expeditiously than one under the current litigation system, but it could also be conducted routinely and privately, among knowledgeable professionals, rather than in the glare of publicity that can accompany litigation.

For quality enhancement, the bill contains provisions that prohibit incompetent physicians and other health care professionals from practicing and that provide immunity from suit for persons reviewing and determining whether treatment was proper; it also requires that state licensing authorities be notified of adverse actions (termination of privileges); and it provides immunity and confidentiality for persons who report incidents of malpractice. This portion of the scheme was enacted into law under a different bill.[29]

Critics of the concept believe that it will result in adverse selection— the provider selecting only the most adverse or certain other malpractice claims for a payment commitment. This practice could occur, but it is not a defect. The tort system does not ensure payment of the most serious cases and does not pay all cases. If there were adverse selection, the most serious cases would be paid and the rest would be no worse off than under present tort law.

The proposal provided a model for the states to consider; the model would have become law with respect to beneficiaries of federal programs if the states did not respond. In my opinion the proposal offers a good alternative to the tort system. Without abandoning the salutary principle that compensation for medical injuries should be based on fault, the proposal encourages providers to compensate patients who are injured by malpractice—and to compensate them quickly and without litigation.

Federal Proposals

Several bills addressing tort reform were introduced in the 100th Congress. No action, including hearings, was taken on any of them, however. A short summary of these bills follows.

The Professional Medical Liability Reform Act of 1987, H.R. 1372, would have established within the U.S. Department of Justice a program to fund the creation and operation of state medical liability arbitration panels. Such panels would have exclusive jurisdiction over nonfederal medical malpractice claims. This bill would have taken medical liability out of the tort system. It would further have abolished the collateral source rule, authorized dismissal of frivolous claims, capped noneconomic damages at $250,000, authorized structured award payments, prescribed procedures and standards to govern judicial review of panel decisions, established a schedule of attorneys' fees, and fixed a statute of limitations.

The National Professional Liability Reform Act of 1987, H.R. 1955, proposed sweeping reforms in state medical practice claims processes, including structured award payments, caps on noneconomic damages, and a schedule of attorneys' fees.

The National Professional Liability Reform Act of 1987, S. 1315, provided for federal incentive grants to encourage state medical malpractice liability reform, including structured damage award payments, caps on noneconomic damages of $250,000, and a schedule of attorneys' fees.

The Health Care Protection Act of 1987, S. 155, encouraged each state to set up medical malpractice screening panels with original and exclusive jurisdiction over such claims. It also limited contingent fees. Another bill, S. 426, provided for limits in the tort system.

The U.S. Department of Health and Human Services recently issued and endorsed a task force report on medical liability and malpractice.[30] This report contains a series of recommended actions to alleviate the current medical malpractice situation. Although it recommends federal involvement in the area of quality control, it does not recommend alternatives to the tort system; rather, it supports state reforms, as discussed above.[31] Moreover, the report develops no strategies for implementation, noting that the department will develop such plans as appropriate.

Provider Proposals

Provider organizations have developed their own proposals. In January 1988 the AMA presented a plan that would substitute an administrative system for the traditional civil jury trial system for medical malpractice claims.[32] Current medical disciplinary boards would be granted expanded, exclusive jurisdiction to hear medical liability disputes; court review would be only on very narrow grounds. Thus, the AMA's proposal would take malpractice out of the judicial tort system. The report further recommends limiting noneconomic damages to $150,000–$170,000, depending on life expectancy; abolishing joint and several liability so that liability is limited to each party's percentage of negligence; establishing a two-year statute of limitations; requiring structured payments on awards above a certain amount; changing the informed consent rule to what a reasonable patient would want to know; abolishing the collateral source rule; and allowing the administrative board to review the reasonableness of attorneys' fees. The report has received much criticism as being unfair to potential claimants.

The AHA has also developed a proposal.[33] This approach focuses on reforms of the tort system. The AHA favors caps on noneconomic damages, abolition of the collateral source rule and of joint and several liability, structured awards, and reduced statutes of limitations.

SUMMARY

Medical malpractice is a complicated issue on which there is no consensus among interest groups. Most agree that the current tort system for handling malpractice claims is costly, time-consuming, and traumatic for victims of malpractice. The best system, however, remains elusive. Until a solution is found, health care costs will continue to escalate and too many victims of malpractice will go uncompensated. Thus far, reforms have merely tinkered with the tort system—none has proven to be really successful. It is time to consider bold solutions that take malpractice out of the tort system and to move consideration of those solutions from academic discussion to legislative action.

REFERENCES AND NOTES

1. In some states the courts and the legislature cannot agree on whether a crisis does or did exist. See *Boucher* v. *Sayeed,* 459 A.2d 87 (R.I. 1983).
2. See Mills, D. H. 1978. Medical insurance feasibility study: A technical summary. Western J. Med. 128:360–365.
3. General Accounting Office (GAO), U.S. Congress. 1987. Medical Malpractice: Characteristics of Claims Closed in 1984. GAO/HRD-87-55. Gaithersburg, Md. To conduct this review, the GAO analyzed data from a random sample of malpractice claims

closed in 1984 by 25 insurers selected from 102 insurers nationwide that wrote a total of $2.3 billion in direct premiums in 1983 for medical malpractice insurance (pp. 2, 14–15). Before this, national data had not been collected since 1978 (p. 14).

4. Ibid., pp. 18–21. The present value of those indemnity payments totals about $2.5 million. Although about 70 percent of the paid claims were for less than $50,000, those claims closed with indemnity payments of more than $250,000 (about 9 percent of paid claims) accounted for about 60 percent of the total indemnity paid (p. 19).

5. Ibid., pp. 23–28, 38, 53–55. Reliable estimates for specific categories of obstetrical errors other than fetal distress could not be determined because of limited data in the sample (p. 23).

6. Ibid., pp. 24–37.

7. Ibid., pp. 36–49. About 88 percent of the economic loss was for anticipated future economic loss (p. 43).

8. General Accounting Office (GAO), U.S. Congress. 1986. Medical Malpractice: Six State Case Studies Show Claims and Insurance Costs Still Rise Despite Reforms. GAO/HRD-87-21. Gaithersburg, Md.

9. Ibid., pp. 2–5.

10. Ibid., pp. 9–20.

11. See, generally, Framme, L. H. 1987. Cinderella: The story of HB 1216. Va. Med. 114:384.

12. See, generally, National Conference of State Legislatures. 1987. Resolving the Liability Insurance Crisis: State Legislative Activities in 1986. Denver.

13. Danzon, P., and L. Lillard. 1982. The Resolution of Medical Malpractice Claims: Modeling and Analysis. Santa Monica, Calif.: Rand Corp. [Hereinafter referred to as the Rand study.]

14. But see *Farley* v. *Engelken,* 241 Kan. 663, 740 P.2d 1058 (Kan. 1987) (abrogation of collateral source rule violated state equal protection clause); see also *Carson* v. *Mauer,* 424 A.2d 825 (N.H. 1980); *Arneson* v. *Olson,* 270 N.W.2d 125 (N.D. 1978).

15. Exclusive control may no longer be a requirement for liability. See *Yabarra* v. *Spangard,* 25 Cal. 2d 486, 154 P.2d 687 (1944).

16. Ibid.

17. Fla. Stat. Ann. § 768.595 (West 1986).

18. Rand study. 1982, pp. 20–21; see note 13.

19. Mass. Gen. Laws Ann. ch. 231, § 601 (West 1984 & Supp. 1987).

20. The New Hampshire Supreme Court held that a contingency fee scale similar to the Massachusetts schedule violates the equal protection clause of the U.S. Constitution. *Carson* v. *Mauer,* 424 A.2d at 839.

21. Rand study. 1982, p. 26; see note 13.

22. *Wisconsin* v. *Wilkie,* 81 Wis. 2d 491, 261 N.W.2d 434 (1978) (upheld a mandatory structured payment plan for awards in excess of $1 million), as opposed to *Carson* v. *Mauer,* 424 A.2d at 838.

23. Because most of the existing caps are set at a relatively high level, however, this reform will have little or no effect in cases involving smaller damage amounts.

24. Rand study. 1982, p. 26; see note 13.

25. *Jones* v. *State Board of Medicine,* 97 Idaho 859, 555 P.2d 399 (1976); *Wright* v. *Central Du Page Hospital Association,* 63 Ill. 2d 313, 347 N.E.2d 736 (1976); *Carson* v. *Mauer; Arneson* v. *Olson; Simon* v. *St. Elizabeth Medical Center,* 3 Ohio Op. 3d 164, 355 N.E.2d 903 (Com. Pl. 1976); *Baptist Hospital of South East Texas* v. *Baber,* 672 S.W.2d 296 (Tex. Civ. App. Beaumont) writ referred without an opinion by the court, 714 S.W.2d 310 (Tex. 1986). A split has recently developed in the Texas appellate courts. Although three appellate courts have found the damage cap unconstitutional, the most recent appellate decision cites a nationwide trend upholding this type of limita-

tion and finds the damage cap constitutional. *Rose* v. *Doctors' Hospital Facilities,* 735 S.W.2d 244 (Tex. Civ. App. Dallas 1987).

26. *Fein* v. *Permanente Medical Group,* 38 Cal. 3d 137, 695 P.2d 665, appeal dismissed, 474 U.S. 892 (1985); *Johnson* v. *St. Vincent Hospital, Inc.,* 273 Ind. 374, 404 N.E.2d 585 (1980); see also *Prendergast* v. *Nelson,* 199 Neb. 97, 256 N.W.2d 657 (1977) (limitation elected prior to treatment upheld).
27. Ibid.
28. See *Carson* v. *Mauer,* 424 A.2d at 839.
29. 42 U.S.C. § 1111 (Supp. IV 1986).
30. U.S. Department of Health and Human Services. 1987. Report of the Task Force on Medical Liability and Malpractice. Washington, D.C.: Government Printing Office.
31. Ibid., pp. 1–53.
32. See American Medical Association—Specialty Society Medical Liability Project. 1988. A Proposed Alternative to the Civil Justice System for Resolving Medical Liability Disputes: A Fault-Based, Administrative System. Chicago.
33. See American Hospital Association, Office of Legal and Regulatory Affairs. 1987. Nontraditional Approaches to the Medical Malpractice Crisis. Chicago.

Index

229

in cesarean section risks, 34
in jury verdicts on malpractice,
168–169, 170–175
in malpractice insurance premiums, 89
in Medicaid reimbursement rates, 2,
88–94
in nurse-midwifery practice, 105
in obstetrical practice patterns, 81, 105,
157
Georgia
changes in obstetrical practice in, 82, 85
jury verdicts on malpractice, 168, 171,
174

Harvard Risk Management Foundation,
36
Hawaii, liability coverage for Medicaid
providers in, 5
Health Care Financing Administration,
53
Health Care Protection Act of 1987, 224
Health care providers, *see* Family and
general practitioners; Nurse-midwives; Obstetrician-gynecologists;
Physicians
Health departments, *see* Public health
agencies/programs
Health insurance
and access to care, 60
Blue Cross, 20, 30
and cesarean deliveries, 30
EFM reimbursement policy, 20
ethical issues, 51
premium increases, 110, 138
reimbursement policies for new technologies, 49, 53
see also Uninsured women
Health maintenance organizations, 48,
118, 196, 197, 205
Hemophilia, 50
High-risk women
characteristics of, 61, 87, 90
EFM use on, 13, 18–19, 20
reduction of care to, 59, 80–83, 87, 90,
137
see also Low-income women; Uninsured
women
Hospitals
closures of obstetrical units, 86
effects of joint and several liability on,
152
emergency room deliveries, 70
exemption from liability for charity
care, 122–123, 133
investor-owned, 30
limits of malpractice coverage, 109
malpractice claims against, by Medicaid
patients, 92
malpractice insurance expenditures by,
154–155
Medicaid deliveries in, 92
not-for-profit, 30
privileges for family practitioners and
nurse-midwives, 69, 109
public, 30, 70

risk management programs, 5
university, *see* Academic medical centers
Hysterectomy, 175, 176–177, 184–186,
188, 189

Idaho, changes in obstetrical practice in,
86, 105
Illinois
changes in obstetrical practice in, 82, 83
jury verdicts on malpractice, 168, 171,
172, 174
malpractice plaintiffs in, 91
Infant mortality
from asphyxia, 17
cesarean deliveries and, 30, 32–33,
34–35
EFM and, 11–13, 15–17
HHS initiative on, 2–3
neonatal intensive care and, 34–35
perinatal causes of, 37
prematurity and, 35
prenatal care and, 3
socioeconomic status and, 35, 87
U.S. rates of, 35, 78
Informed consent, 23, 101–103, 116,
146–147
Institute of Medicine, Council on Health
Care Technology, 12, 21
Insurance, *see* Health insurance; Malpractice insurance
Insurance industry
ethical issues involving, 51
regulation of, 215
taxes on, to fund no-fault compensation,
126, 129–130, 196
underwriting practices, 5
see also Malpractice insurance
Intensive care, neonatal, 3, 12–13, 15, 16,
34–35
Ireland
EFM clinical trials, 12–15
PKU screening in, 45

Johns Hopkins University, 44, 47, 165
Johnson, Kirk, 162, 163
Joint underwriting associations, 109
Jury verdicts
ability of juries to evaluate medical
testimony, 138, 190
on abortion cases, 175, 176, 183–186,
189
by cause of injury, 179–184, 186–189,
191
by class of injury, 180–181, 184–185
collateral source rule and, 218
consistency of, 138, 156–157, 187
emotional basis for, 4, 23, 98, 150
filed cases resulting in, 167, 195
geographic distribution of, 168–169,
170–175
on hysterectomy cases, 175, 176–177,
184–186, 188, 189
influence on out-of-court settlements,
163–164, 167–169, 176, 207